ADVANCE PRAISE

Early feedback from Goodreads reviewers

"A beautifully written personal account of survival... This is not a misery memoir—it's a story about survival and a refusal to let what happened define the rest of her life."

— LOUISE

"A story from the spectrum that confronts a notorious failure of the criminal justice system... Highly recommended."

— SHANE

"A wonderfully written, heartbreaking recounting of the rollercoaster people experience after traumatic events... Definitely worth reading."

— LIZ

"An honest account of a horrific, lived experience and the true meaning of trauma—how it affects everyday life. I think every health care professional should read it."

— ANNMARIE

NOT THE PERFECT VICTIM

Not the Perfect Victim

A Memoir of Surviving Sexual Violence, a Late
Autism Diagnosis, and the Fight for Justice

BY

ANNA KAHILL

First edition

ISBN 978-1-0682903-0-5

Contents

In loving memory of my beautiful mother

Missing you more than words can express.

I love you, and I will carry you with me forever.

Before the Story Begins

Trigger Warning

This book contains content that may be distressing or upsetting to some readers. It includes accounts of sexualised violence, trauma, and other sensitive topics. Reader discretion is strongly advised.

Please be aware that the experiences, thoughts, feelings, and opinions shared in this book are deeply personal and unique to my own journey. While I may express sentiments that I feel could resonate with other victims or survivors of trauma, it is important to understand that everyone's experiences are different. The way in which we process, understand, and react to trauma varies from person to person, and not all survivors will share the same emotions or viewpoints.

I do not intend to speak for all victims, survivors or autistic women, as we all have individual differences, just like anyone else. However, there may be themes throughout this book that are universally relatable to those who have lived through trauma. These themes, such as the complex emotions tied to healing and the pursuit of justice, are not one-size-fits-all but may still echo across diverse experiences of pain and recovery.

I write this book for myself, sharing my truth as I have lived it, but I also stand in solidarity with others who have experienced similar suffering, regardless of the differences in our stories. Our collective voices, though varied, can hold power, and it is my hope that in sharing my journey, others may find a sense of connection and, perhaps, a path towards healing, if that is their choice.

If you or someone you know may be affected by the subjects discussed in this book, please take care when reading and seek support if needed. At the end of this book, you will find suggestions for support resources.

Disclaimer

Truthful, But Not Literal

This memoir is a work of non-fiction based on the author's personal experiences. Some names, locations, and identifying details have been changed or omitted to protect the privacy of individuals and to ensure confidentiality. Certain individuals are composites or anonymised. While the events described are truthful to the best of the author's memory, some details may have been adjusted for the sake of clarity, narrative flow, or to respect the privacy of others. Every effort has been made to preserve the emotional truth of the story while safeguarding the identities of those involved. Where ambiguity exists, it is intentional – this book is not intended to accuse, but to heal.

Legal and Investigative Context

This memoir includes references to a personal traumatic event that was reported to the police as a non-recent crime, but the matter was subsequently closed. In the event that the case is reopened or further investigation is pursued, the author wishes to make clear that this work is not intended to influence or interfere with any legal proceedings. Any resemblance to actual persons, living or dead, is purely coincidental. Furthermore, reliving and writing about the trauma may have brought additional clarity or detail that was not previously voiced during the reporting processes.

Intent to Avoid Harm

The author has taken reasonable steps to ensure that the contents of this work do not cause harm or distress to others. The purpose of this book is to offer personal insight and reflection, and it should not be interpreted as a statement on any specific legal case or matter.

Reconstructed Dialogue and Scenes

While every effort has been made to portray events, conversations, and interactions as accurately as possible, the dialogue and scenes in this book are based on the author's best recollection. In some cases, conversations have been reconstructed, paraphrased, or condensed for clarity and narrative flow. Although not all dialogue is presented word for word, the essence and truth of the experiences have been preserved. No contemporaneous notes or recordings were made at the time of the original events.

Personal Experience and not Medical Advice

As a healthcare professional, the author also wishes to clarify that any references to medical treatments, psychological therapies, or non-conventional or complementary approaches are shared solely from a personal perspective. This memoir is not intended to offer medical advice or professional guidance.

Nothing within these pages should be interpreted as a recommendation, diagnosis, or endorsement of any specific treatment, therapy, medication, or intervention. The experiences described reflect the author's individual journey and may not be appropriate or effective for others. Readers should always consult a qualified medical or mental health professional before making decisions regarding their own health or care. Any actions taken based on the content of this book are the sole responsibility of the reader.

The views expressed are entirely the author's own and do not represent the official stance of any organisation, employer, or regulatory body with which they are affiliated. This work is written in a personal, not professional, capacity.

Dialogue and Therapy Depictions Notice

This memoir includes scenes of dialogue and interaction that are reconstructed from the author's memory, emotional experience, and creative interpretation. These conversations — including those with medical professionals, friends, and therapists — are paraphrased or reimagined and used as a literary device to reflect emotional truth. They should not be taken as verbatim or as an exact record of what was said by any individual.

The two therapists referred to in this book are represented under fictional names and are composite, anonymised characters created to protect their privacy. These therapy depictions are not clinical records and should not be interpreted as therapeutic advice, professional commentary, or evidence of any therapist's involvement or participation.

No therapist has reviewed, contributed to, or been consulted about the writing or publication of this memoir. All portrayals are solely the author's own.

A Snapshot in Time

The thoughts, opinions, and reflections shared in this memoir represent the author's personal experiences and understanding at the time of writing and publishing. The author acknowledges that, as their journey of healing, therapy, and personal growth continues, their views and interpretations may evolve. What is expressed in this book is true to the author's feelings and insights at the moment of publication; however, over time, their perspective may change, and their current understanding may not reflect how they feel or think in the future. This book is a snapshot of the author's experience, and they recognise that healing is an ongoing process — one that may lead to new insights and changes in perspective.

Prologue

I didn't know the moment my voice was stolen. But I remember the first time I tried to scream and nothing came out.

In criminal cases in the UK, when a defendant is found guilty, the victim is offered the opportunity to provide an impact statement. With the case closed and no trial forthcoming, I turned to sharing my story in this book as my form of an impact statement. I am a victim of a heinous crime, and this book is my impact statement.

Unfortunately, due to our outdated, prehistoric criminal justice system – where disproportionate weight is often given to the *he* in a *he-said, she-said* argument – I was not given the opportunity to take my case to court, and therefore not offered the chance to officially share, within the criminal justice system, the impact that this crime has had on me. Consequently, I am empowering myself by reclaiming my voice through the publication of my story.

It has taken me well over a decade, my mum's death from cancer, and a psychoanalytical journey to finally use the word *rape* to describe what happened to me. It took me even longer to understand that it was not my fault.

Once I was ready to speak, around the time I reported the rape, I struggled to remain silent. After fifteen years of keeping this secret, and enduring two more within the criminal justice process, I finally release myself from that struggle.

Maya Angelou's words especially ring true: "There is no greater agony than bearing an untold story inside you."[1]

---

1 Maya Angelou, *I Know Why the Caged Bird Sings* (New York: Random House, 2009)

This impact statement is told through the lens of my therapeutic journey – my life before and after the rape. My story explores themes of trauma mistaken for identity, late diagnosis of autism, masking and unmasking, motherhood, and the many pitfalls of the criminal justice system.

As you read through my story, you may begin to question your own. I encourage you to do so.

However, if you choose to explore the depths of your own heart and mind, make sure you are strong enough to navigate them. Many people struggle to do this without support – I know I did. It's important to feel safe and accepted if you are to confront the lurking shadows within.

"…it's not for us to have shame – it's for them."

GISÈLE PELICOT[2]

---

2 Willsher, Kim. "French Court Acquits Men Accused of Raping Gisele Pelicot in Landmark Consent Case." *The Guardian*, 23 October 2024, https://www. theguardian.com/world/2024/oct/23/gisele-pelicot-rape-trial-france-court.

Author's Note on Language, Allegation and Identification

In this book, I refer to a man as "the man who raped me". This language reflects my lived experience, my memory, and my testimony. I reported this man to the police in 2023, and I stand by what I told them – that I was raped. These words are not used lightly. They come from years of trauma, dissociation, silence, and eventually, the painful process of healing and truth-telling.

I am aware that authors are often advised, for legal protection, to use softer or more legally cautious phrases – such as "the man I allege raped me", or "what he did felt like rape" – especially when no criminal conviction exists. This advice is rooted in defamation law, which can penalize survivors for speaking plainly about their experiences. But I have chosen not to soften or dilute my words.

To describe what happened to me in any other way would be a betrayal of my truth. I will not place legal caution above my own lived reality. I was raped. That is what I told the police. That is what I told my therapist. That is what I am telling you.

The man who raped me was not someone I knew. There was no warning, no history – he wasn't part of my story until he tore into it. If, at times, the reader feels like I did know him, that is only a reflection of the trauma's aftermath and the years I spent processing his impact. My emotional responses to seeing him again, or recalling what followed, are not evidence of a prior relationship – only of what it means to survive something so violating.

At the time of publication, no charges have been brought against the man I refer to, and the allegations described have not been proven in court. The man denies wrongdoing. My use of the word "rape" reflects my experience – not a legal verdict.

Additionally, some readers may feel they recognise individuals in this book – particularly where old friendships or shared histories are part of the narrative. But let me be clear: this is not about exposing or accusing any one person. I have changed names and, where needed, adjusted contextual details to protect privacy. This book is not about identifying others. It is about telling the truth of what happened to me, and how silence shaped my story. If you believe you know who I'm referring to, you don't – because this is not their story. It's mine.

This is my story, as I experienced and remember it. It is my truth.

Trauma

The central focus of this book is the impact of trauma. However, I'm conscious of the widespread misuse of this term in modern society, which makes me somewhat apprehensive about using it, even in relation to my own experience of sexualised violence. Because of this, I feel compelled to share the correct definition of trauma.

The word *trauma* originates from the Greek term for "wound".[3] Trauma *is* the wound; it is not the event that causes it. Medical definitions of trauma include exposure to "actual or threatened death, serious injury, or sexualised violence"[4] or "any disturbing experience that results in significant fear, helplessness, dissociation, confusion, or other disruptive feelings intense enough to have a long-lasting negative effect on a person's attitudes, behaviour, and other aspects of functioning".[5] Another definition describes trauma as "a distressing event or events so extreme or intense that they overwhelm a person's ability to cope, resulting in lasting negative impact".[6]

Despite being a medical term, the word *trauma* is now used casually and frequently in everyday language. People often describe themselves as "traumatised" by a film, a stressful commute, a hurtful remark, or a difficult relationship – although it's worth

---

3 Kolaitis, G., and Olff, M. "Psychotraumatology in Greece." *European Journal of Psychotraumatology*, vol. 8, supp. 4, 29 September 2017, article 1351757. https://doi.org/10.1080/20008198.2017.1351757.

4 *The Diagnostic and Statistical Manual of Mental Disorders*, Fifth Edition, Text Revision (DSM-5-TR). American Psychiatric Association.

5 American Psychological Association. "Trauma." *APA Dictionary of Psychology*. https://dictionary.apa.org/trauma

6 UK Trauma Council. "What Is Trauma?" https://uktraumacouncil.org/trauma/trauma?cn-reloaded=1

noting that abusive relationships *can* be traumatic. Still, many of these examples are not truly traumatic. They are upsetting, yes, but not trauma in the clinical or psychological sense. The widespread misuse of the word dilutes its meaning and undermines its seriousness.

Trauma can vary significantly, both in its cause and in how it affects each individual. Victims of sexualised violence – such as rape – often experience trauma in ways that are distinct from victims of other forms of violence.[7]

"Trauma doesn't build a strong person; you cannot frame hurt and pain that way. Life isn't made better by suffering, can we stop this propaganda?"[8]

---

7 Schnittker, Jason. "What Makes Sexual Violence Different? Comparing the Effects of Sexual and Non-Sexual Violence on Psychological Distress." *SSM – Mental Health*, vol. 2, 2022, article 100115. https://doi.org/10.1016/j.ssmmh.2022.100115.

8 Brown, Amanda. *No Peace Until He's Dead*. Merrion Press, 23 February 2024.

Bath of Silence

Seated behind the steering wheel for the first time in a very long time – dry-mouthed, body rigid, and staring intensely at the modest-looking entrance of the private clinic – I wait, anxiously, to see who this therapist David is.

I've been sitting here for at least thirty minutes before my appointment. My anticipatory anxiety rises until a lump forms in my throat. I'm ready to ignite the engine and accelerate out of there. I seriously contemplate leaving when a smartly dressed man, old enough to be my father, steps out of the entrance and raises his arm, signalling me to come in.

I open the car door, and just as my black heels hit the tarmac, a gentle September breeze lifts the premature grey patches of my hair from my pale face. My tiny, underweight frame, clothed entirely in black, makes its way towards the man. I try to hide my awkwardness by deliberately injecting a bit of confidence into my stride.

He greets me with a cool demeanour and a neutral expression. *Thank God I have to wear a COVID face mask,* I think. *At least that way, I don't have to force a smile back.*

David leads the way, and with every step, I dread more and more what is to come.

He invites me into a small consultation room. It's nothing special – actually, it's a little disappointing – though I'm not sure what I was expecting. Once inside, he suggests I remove my mask. I realise there is no hiding from this man.

Sitting opposite each other, I wait for David to speak. But he doesn't.

In the silence, we stare at each other, and I feel utterly uncomfortable.

What the fuck is happening here? Why the fuck is he not speaking?
My eyes, framed in heavy black eyeliner – much too dark for my complexion – can no longer meet his. I most certainly cannot remain at ease in this bath of silence.

And just when my body can no longer conceal the discomfort, he speaks.

Thank fuck. What a relief.

That day marked the beginning of my healing journey. Analysis had begun.

Over the weeks, I came to understand that the silence – the space between my words, the space between the therapist and me – was exactly what David was observing. The things I wasn't saying were the things he gently inquired about. He read my body language as easily as reading words off a page.

I began to speak aloud for the first time about things I had never dared to talk about – perhaps not even dared to think about fully.

In between sessions, I began unravelling the tangles that tormented my inner world. And in all that unravelling, I travelled back and forth through my life.

I came face-to-face with myself in a new way. I let her – the inner me – speak for the first time.

Her story, and what she says, will be told. Because what ~~he-says~~ *she-says* matters too.

Walk with her. Run with her. Sit with her. Laugh with her. Cry.

Maybe you'll meet yourself, too, as we run into the darkness together.

The World As I Knew It

Childhood And Family

Chapter 1: Home

"Home is not a place, it's a feeling."

— CECELIA AHERN

I was a quiet child, number four out of five siblings. For five whole years, I was the youngest, the baby of the house. Life was good in that role, but everything changed , when a surprise baby arrived: our youngest sister. According to Mum, when she was born, my nose was knocked out of joint. I was no longer the baby – I was suddenly the middle of three girls.

From that point on, if I was lucky, I got called by my name. More often, I was simply referred to as "Number 4", based on my birth order. My dad had affectionate pet names for us three girls, which I'll use throughout this memoir: Toodles, Petals, and Cuddles, in that order. The boys had their own nicknames too. One of mine was "Mum's shadow", because I followed her wherever she went. That bond lasted well into early adulthood. I was rarely seen without her. My mum was my safe place.

We grew up a family of seven in a three-bedroom, semi-detached house in Brackenhill Park, a council estate in Newry, Northern Ireland. Sharing a small house with six others was a full-on sensory experience, often bordering on daily drama. There was the pain of holding "it" in while waiting for the bathroom, versus the anxiety of sitting on the loo while the handle jiggled frantically from the other side. The smell of toast would drift enticingly from the grill – or later, the toaster – only to be met with disappointment when someone else had nabbed the first batch. The sound of the kettle boiling, then reboiling, was almost drowned out by squabbles about who had been in the kitchen first.

At one point, things got so competitive that the eldest two started bringing the kettle upstairs the night before, plugging it in beside the bed. They took turns each week making tea for each other from the comfort of their beds. To this day, I still don't know where they kept the milk.

Weekends were no exception. Sunday mornings brought the aroma of chicken roasting in the oven and the clatter of kitchen utensils as Dad prepared Sunday dinner, giving Mum a well-earned break from weekday cooking. My scrawny frame, draped in oversized pyjamas, would clamber down the stairs, following the smell to its source. The kitchen was usually in chaos – pots, pans, potato skins, and knives strewn everywhere. It looked as if the chicken had been free-ranging in the kitchen before it ended up in the oven.

Dad was a great cook, and Mum preferred it when he took charge of the meals. But she was much better at tidying as she went, so it was always obvious who had cooked, based on the state of the kitchen. Despite the mess and the strange fusion of roasting chicken and toasting bread, the house still felt like a home. I found peace in the familiar. The clutter faded into the background as I sat at the table eating breakfast, listening to the sound of Mum turning the pages of the Sunday papers that Dad had picked up after Mass. The two of them would sit together, solving crossword puzzles, with Mum reading the clues aloud.

With seven people under one roof, our home was always bustling and noisy. Whether it was the hiss of the iron as Mum tackled another mountain of laundry, the thud of someone tripping over the 50-kilogram sack of spuds by the back door, the rhythmic sound of potatoes being peeled for dinner, or the constant chorus of siblings bickering – it was alive. We got on each other's nerves, yes, but we also shared belly-aching laughter and endless inside jokes.

While the sensory overload could be exhausting, there was comfort in its consistency. It was a home full of people, noise, and emotion. But above all, it was a home founded on love.

Chapter 2: Doors Unlocked

While our home in Brackenhill Park didn't differ much from many other council estates in the North of Ireland, the same couldn't be said for the towns themselves. The major distinctions between towns were primarily defined by religion. Some were predominantly Catholic, others Protestant, and a few had a mix of both. With religion so deeply intertwined with politics here, even now, the news remains dominated by seemingly trivial "green" (Catholic) versus "orange" (Protestant) issues, sometimes stretching right through to sectarian violence and hate crimes. These tensions were always more pronounced in mixed towns.

As kids, we became desensitised to the daily news of violence. Unless something happened in Newry, we hardly paid attention. And since Newry was predominantly Catholic, there wasn't much local "trouble" to entertain or concern us. When something *did* happen, it was a big deal.

In my younger years, I remember the police knocking on our door in the middle of the night, instructing the whole family to move to the back of the house. They suspected a bomb had been left in the commercial yard near our housing estate. My parents dragged mattresses into their bedroom so we could all sleep together for the rest of the night. While Mum and Dad could have done without the disruption, for us kids, it was great craic. The whispers and giggles under the covers that night were much to our parents' dismay.

A few years later, a suspicious device was found at the entrance to our estate. I'll never forget standing among the other children, watching the bomb disposal robot trundle towards the object. Without wishing harm or damage, I felt a strange excitement at the possibility of the bomb exploding. Fortunately, it never did – just another scare.

Despite the rarity of local incidents, and the national news often falling on deaf ears, there was a stubborn and sometimes aggressive determination in Northern Ireland to remind us of the underlying tensions. From our house in the valley of Newry, we had a view of a British Army base. It loomed from Cloughoge, nestled awkwardly beside the beautiful and enchanting Ring of Gullion.

The regular ascension of military helicopters and their routine journeys across the airspace above our home created a familiar soundscape. The rhythmic beating of their blades became part of our daily life. The choppers would circle directly overhead, their thumping rattling our windows and doors. Despite the noise, we could still fall asleep to the sound.

Maybe we were unknowingly lulled into a meditative state each night, immersed in something like a binaural beat. Or maybe I just refused to acknowledge the fear they tried to instil in the people of Newry.

As part of their routine, the choppers would land in an abandoned field close to our estate that we called *The Hilly Field*, now a housing development known as Maple Grove. I remember the rush of adrenaline as we sprinted there with uncontainable excitement to see the helicopters and soldiers land. We were gutted if we missed a landing or take-off. To this day, I still have no idea why the British Army regularly made those regular trips from Cloughoge to The Hilly Field. They never seemed to do anything while they were there. No sooner had they landed than they were gone again.

As a curious child, I had a thousand questions. I hadn't realised they were British soldiers until Mum and Dad told me – I'd just assumed they were Irish. When I found out they weren't, it opened up a floodgate. It was probably the first time I was ever educated, albeit briefly, on Irish history.

"Why are there no Irish soldiers landing here?" I'd ask, in every variation I could think of. The feelings of injustice that rose in my belly were overwhelming. I fired off questions with barely a breath in between. It felt like that injustice had been trapped in my DNA for generations, finally finding a way out through my voice. It was hard to comprehend how one country could march into another and claim it as its own.

That same feeling of injustice resurfaced every Friday night – our homemade fish and chip night – when my siblings stole chips from my plate. They might say I did the same, but I genuinely don't remember doing so. Counting our chips became normal. Spuds were, and still are, sacred in the Irish family. I suppose we're protective of them because of the intergenerational trauma left behind by the Great Famine of the 1800s.

We never truly got over our political past, especially when it came to our food. During the famine, while the Irish starved, our produce was shipped to England.[9] It was genocide. Thousands of families perished, including those who fled on the transatlantic famine ships – *coffin ships*, as they were known. The conditions were inhumane both on land and at sea. We were dehumanised as a people and as a nation. So, when I kept tabs on the number of chips on my plate, it wasn't just sibling rivalry. It was the echo of a famine wound still felt in our bones.

The trauma we carried in Northern Ireland wasn't mine alone. *The Troubles* were the direct result of centuries of conflict: British versus Irish, Taig versus Hun, Catholic versus Protestant. Still green versus orange.

The news in Newry never seemed as saturated with violence as places like Belfast. In the grand scheme, Newry felt like a safe place to grow up. Despite the presence of armed soldiers and choppers overhead, we left our doors unlocked at night. Neigh-

---

9 Institute for Global Health and Migration. "Learn." IGMH. https://www.ighm.org/learn.html

bours let themselves in during the day. We played freely on the street, wandered into other neighbourhoods, and walked up the main road to the shop we called *The Nifty* – all without our parents worrying.

That started to change in the 2000s, as Newry expanded and grew. But for most of my childhood, Newry seemed safe.

Chapter 3: Blackberry Jam

Friendships were always a challenge for me. I played with kids in the neighbourhood and made friends in school, but I never seemed to form lasting connections. I struggled to grasp whatever it was I was supposed to understand – their jokes, their timing, their kind of humour. Some friendships felt wholesome but were short-lived and, in hindsight, questionable. I had, and have no real social group – no shared circles, no long-standing tribe. Few, if any, of those friends knew each other. This book reflects how those connections impacted me personally, but no single person could know the full picture – not even them.

One particular friendship lingered from childhood into early adulthood – a rare thread in an otherwise scattered social web. We felt like kindred spirits at times, inseparable in childhood, but that closeness shifted and fractured in ways I still don't fully understand. We whispered secrets and laughed at nonsense, but the connection, in hindsight, feels harder to define than I once believed. It was not until my thirties that I discovered the painful truth: this friendship for life was nothing more than an illusionary friendship. *I will later refer to this friend only in the abstract.* But I also had another close friendship – one I still look back on fondly. Keira. Somehow, we just got each other. Like *my other friend*, our bond was obsessive in that childhood way, but with Keira, it always felt lighter. We could play for hours, days, even weeks on end – until the intensity grew too much, and we needed a break. Our rhythm had a natural cycle: together, then apart, then back together again. This continued for years, until our early teens, when life began pulling us in different directions.

During those intense stretches, we were inseparable. We played at each other's homes and in the local play park. The parks in the 1990s weren't what they are now. Safety wasn't much of a concern – concrete or tarmac underfoot, rusty metal frames, splintery wooden beams. Burning our arses on the metal slide in summer was just the price we paid for a few seconds of thrill. And in the rain, which was often, we'd wait for someone else to go down the slide first and dry it off for the rest of us.

Our real adventures happened "up the rocks" – a patch of wild wasteland with a small quarry tucked behind the local play park. It's all fenced off now, probably after the Newry and Mourne Council finally realised it wasn't the safest place for kids. But back then, we didn't care. We fought our way through bracken and thorns, collecting scratches like badges. The brush whipped our legs and arms, but we pushed on, balancing along muddy tracks with steep drops beside us, leaping from boulder to boulder, climbing the quarry like explorers in a forgotten land.

We talked about everything and nothing as we wandered the rocks, giggling until our sides ached. We could smell summer before it arrived – the buzz of bees, the hum of insects, the warm September air that comes just before the first real winds of autumn, and then the early darkness of winter rolling in. We breathed it all in, fumbled through the bush, and ran wild through the green. Kids today don't know what they're missing.

As we got older, the rocks gave way to the Greenan Walk – a local route everyone in the neighbourhood knew. It's a walk that links the old Warrenpoint Road – the *Point Road* – with the lush Greenan Road, past the open greens of Commons Hall Road, looping back through the town by St. Mary's Church, or sometimes shortcutting through Commons Way to rejoin the nearby housing estates or onwards to the Point Road again. To this day, I still do the Greenan.

One autumn, Keira and I hiked the Greenan and harvested blackberries, stripping the bramble bushes bare. We were going to make a few quid selling homemade blackberry jam. With sticky fingers and bursting bags, we brought the berries back to my house. Mum gently discouraged us – her kitchen was barely functional, and she could already picture the mess – but she didn't stop us either.

We washed the blackberries and dumped them into a giant pot, piling in sugar and water – none of it measured, of course – then turned the gas on full. At that point, Keira bailed, and I was left alone with the task. I carried on enthusiastically, until something stomach-churning put an abrupt end to the plan – and to my love of blackberries.

I remember glancing into the pot to check if the jam was forming. It had only just started heating up when I noticed small dark specks floating on the surface. I leaned in for a closer look.

What I saw turned my stomach: maggots. Dozens of them, weaving their way out of the blackberries as the pot warmed. I froze in disgust. I could not make blackberry and *maggot* jam, and I certainly couldn't sell it to anyone in good conscience. I dumped the entire pot.

Dad, never liking the idea of waste and tried to save some of it. With a classic daddy joke, he said, "Ah sure, the extra protein'll do us good!"

After that, I didn't eat another blackberry for years, well into adulthood. And to this day, I still avoid blackberry jam.

Chapter 4: Tartan Trousers

The making of blackberry and maggot jam was not my only adventure. Though friendships were often a challenge for me, they weren't impossible. I'll never forget the craic with the girls at the back of Brackenhill Park.

One memory stands out from my pre-teen years: trying to sleep in a wooden shed that had been purpose-built by one of their dads. The idea of it was thrilling, but the cold seeped into our bones, and my bony arse had enough of the hard wooden floor – even with a sleeping bag underneath. Eventually, we retreated to the living room, but not a wink of sleep was had. Even though I sat quietly and shyly while the girls chatted and laughed until dawn, I still felt included. I made my way home as the sun rose, exhausted but content that I had managed to stay the night. I think that was my first ever sleepover, though I might be wrong. Every sleepover outside my own home brought the same nerves. I was always a quiet bag of tension when sleeping anywhere unfamiliar.

I was an odd child, though I couldn't pinpoint how or why, and I didn't know how to communicate the differences I felt. Still, the girls seemed inclusive and kind. I remember them inviting me to St. Mary's Youth Club disco one Friday evening. I had never been to the youth club before – never even been to a disco. Embarrassed, my cheeks flushed red as I told them I couldn't go; I didn't know how to dance. A couple of them laughed and said they'd teach me. I wish I'd taken them up on that offer. Being included meant the world to me, but I was too timid to dance in public and too self-conscious to learn from my peers.

But I wasn't always a stranger to singing or dancing. The '90s were the Spice Girls era, when "girl power" seemed to unite us all.

Inspired by that magic, I formed my own girl band – a sisterhood of shared dreams and promised fame.

One girl from the back of Brackenhill Park was a core member. We spent hours in her house, practising, messing about, and planning our rise to stardom. The girl power we felt in Brackenhill Park extended into St. Clare's Primary School, a large, crumbling convent school on Castle Street that was demolished in 2024. We had a school-based band, too, with other classmates, whom I still remember fondly.

But girl power, it turns out, didn't always extend to me.

The girls were also friends with some others from Tullagh View, an estate that adjoined the back of Brackenhill Park. I didn't know the Tullagh View girls very well, but I admired one of them from afar. She seemed like their ringleader – taller than me, possibly older, effortlessly stylish, and radiating a kind of confidence I couldn't even fake. I had barely exchanged a word with her, but I was captivated. Her presence, her voice, even her clothes fascinated me.

I remember one particular day she wore a pair of tartan trousers that made a lasting impression. I loved them. I went home and told Mum I really wanted a pair of tartan trousers. Money was tight, so she suggested I wait until Christmas and get them as part of my Christmas clothes.

Weeks passed. Then, on one of our Christmas shopping trips, we went to Tammy Girl – the trendiest store in Newry back then – in the Buttercrane Shopping Centre. The clothes in Tammy Girl sparkled with the charm of the Spice Girls themselves. And there, hanging on a rail, was a pair of tartan trousers just like the ones I had admired. I told Mum those were the ones I wanted. She asked me several times if I was sure and suggested we look around a bit more, but I knew my mind. I needed those trousers.

I wore them all through Christmas and into the new year. Then, one day, I went to the back of Brackenhill Park to catch up with the girls. They happened to be meeting the Tullagh View girls as well, right where the two estates met. I hadn't seen the ringleader girl in a while, and when she spotted me wearing my tartan trousers, she scoffed. Though I cannot remember her exact words, it was something close to: "What's she doing here? Look at the state of her trousers. I wouldn't be seen dead hanging around with someone in those."

If it's possible to feel like all eyes are on you while also being completely invisible, that's what I felt in that moment. My face flushed with mortification. It was like I had been forced to carry a shame that didn't belong to me, and yet I was made to believe it had always been mine.

What happened next is a blur, but a couple of memories always stand out. I recall one of the girls quietly saying, "That's awful," in my defence. But I turned on my heels and walked away. That's the last time I remember hanging out with the girls at the back of Brackenhill Park.

For weeks – no, for years – I replayed that moment in my mind, trying to understand why someone would mock me for wearing the same trousers they once wore. I didn't understand then. It wasn't until adulthood that I started to unravel why I might have been singled out like that.

Girl power didn't feel very real that day. It felt fragile, conditional – something that didn't quite extend to quiet, odd girls like me.

Loneliness started to take root in my heart and grew quietly over time, watered by moments like that one. And it was that loneliness that made me even more vulnerable.

Children can be cruel sometimes.

Teen Years and Early Independence

Chapter 5: Teenage Rebellion

The transition from childhood to adulthood felt like crossing a bridge – from my quiet, shy self to someone livelier, more fun. It was a kind of coming-of-age we all experience in our own way.

I discovered a real love for music, and I loved dancing to it even more. The thump of the beats moved through my body as I let the rhythm take over. No one needed to teach me – I could just do it, and it was freeing. Dancing under the mystical disco lights that sliced through smoky air awakened something in me.

While some teenagers discreetly drank vodka from bottles strapped to their thighs with sticky tape, I was one of the ones dancing on tables at Caesars nightclub, just across the border from Newry, near the Carrickdale. I didn't need alcohol; music was my drug. Yet somehow, word got back to my mother that I was "off my face" on drink. Our neighbour's first cousin had seen me, and, with what felt like smug satisfaction, told my mum she should have a word, as though eager to cast me as a disappointment.

My mum came straight to me and asked if the drinking story was true. I told her no, and she believed me. I hadn't touched a drop. In my early teens, drinking still felt like a leap too far. I wanted rebellion, sure, but dancing on tables was the height of mine. Sneaking sips of alcohol? That felt like a rebellion too far. Something always stopped me: the rules.

It wasn't until closer to my eighteenth birthday that alcohol even became a curiosity. By then, I had already slipped into a few over-18s clubs, hiding behind a full mask of foundation, thick on my skin, and layers of fake tan that left an orange tinge on everything I touched. When I went out with Toodles and her friends, I became one of them – a girl in her twenties, easily lost in the crowd and the flicker of strobe lights.

Outings with girls my own age were more nerve-racking. We held our breath in the queue, each second ticking past with pounding hearts. Sometimes, we were turned away, and the sting of rejection clung to us the whole walk home. But when we got in, it was magic.

The music drowned out thought as the DJ's beats thumped through our chests. Clothes clung to our backs with sweat, hair stuck to our necks, and we inhaled second-hand smoke like it was nothing. But none of that mattered. The sense of aliveness – the spinning lights, the energy, the craic – made our whole week. Some of those nights were among the best of my teenage life.

Even as I tasted rebellion, something uneasy stirred inside me. I liked security. I liked rules. I liked knowing what to expect. That comfort extended to everything – school, religion, routine. To others – siblings, classmates, even neighbours' parents – I must have seemed like a goody two-shoes. But for me, it wasn't about being good. It was about feeling safe. Rules were a shield against the unknown.

I did come out of my shell in some ways, but I still clung to the familiar. I was shy about starting conversations, afraid of rejection, uneasy in new places. Having *a special friend* – the one who declared I was their closest person – made me feel anchored. It gave me a sense of connection, of safety. Though I now know it was just an illusion.

Like most teenagers, I was vulnerable to the emotional toxins of the world around me. But some of us are more absorbent than others. I didn't yet know how different I was. I assumed everyone felt things the same way I did – that we were all just figuring it out together. But we weren't. My difference clung to me like a quiet shadow, especially in friendships.

What I longed for was a girl gang. A tight-knit circle. A lifelong sisterhood. The kind of friends who grew together through all stages of life, passed notes in class, got ready together on Friday nights, and promised secrets would never leave the group. I wanted that bond, that safety net, and the unconditional loyalty I saw in impenetrable school cliques and on TV.

But I didn't have it. And without it, I felt exposed in ways I couldn't yet understand.

Loneliness made its home in me quietly, like dust collecting in corners. It wasn't loud, but it was persistent.

Chapter 6: The Off-Licence

Apart from the occasional social outing, I spent much of my time from childhood through to adulthood either buried in books or practising the violin – loudly, relentlessly, and often to everyone's dismay. But studying and screeching my way through the scales wasn't all I wanted to do. I longed for independence – and the pocket money that came with a part-time job.

I was about thirteen when I got my first job in an ice cream shop. That summer was spent dashing in and out of the walk-in freezer, the icy air hitting my arms before giving way to the heat of scrubbing sticky floors and surfaces. My eyes lit up, scooping creamy balls of mint and chocolate, often sneaking a taste of new or favourite flavours. Just as I was getting the hang of it – learning the art of banter and earning £2.50 per hour – the job ended. The manager decided to stop employing underage, cash-in-hand workers. I was devastated, but even more determined to try again.

The following year, I landed a job in the kitchen of a restaurant for £2 an hour. Friday evenings and all-day Saturdays meant sweating over chip pans and meat grills, the oily heat clinging to my skin. The novelty faded quickly. After a few months, I'd had enough. I came home each week with oil-soaked hair, reeking of overcooked grease, and hands blistered from burns. My mum was worried. I was done. I waited patiently until I was of legal age to look again.

At sixteen, I tried a few different jobs. Some didn't work out, but others did. That's when I first noticed my social challenges surfacing at work. Even so, there were jobs I truly enjoyed. For two years, I worked as Santa's helper in the Buttercrane Shopping Centre. I'd stand in the middle of the centre with a bunch of helium balloons, the strings squeaking through my fingers as I fished out the balloon of choice for some impatient kid. I bounced from customer to customer, one hand full of balloons, the other collecting cash. The crinkle of paper notes, the jingle of coins in my bum bag. I practised banter. I got better at it. I chatted with parents, colleagues, and even the security guards.

I also took on a temporary position as a Christmas employee in a busy retail shop. That's where I finally came out of my shell. The staff came from various backgrounds and ages, and I found my place among them. I understood the jokes – and even made a few of my own. I thrived when we were given sales targets for product insurance. Exceeding those targets felt amazing. I learned a hard lesson later when a senior staff member took credit for my sales, but I still managed to hold down both jobs while preparing for national exams. I thrived on the busyness of it all.

Not long before my eighteenth birthday, I started working in an off-licence. I was paid £5 an hour, working during the holidays and covering weekend and evening shifts while at university. I had no prior knowledge of alcohol. I didn't know that red wine should be kept at room temperature. I couldn't tell beer from cider. I didn't know the difference between spirits. But I soon learned. Toodles joined me there, and we had great craic working side by side.

But the real banter came from the customers. An off-licence attracts a different kind of crowd than shopping centres or retail shops. Alcohol brings people together – for celebrations, commiserations, adversity, sickness, and death. Customers came from every part of Newry society. Some were regulars, so predictable that we had their orders ready before they even spoke. Others were occasional, but still familiar. We saw hen and stag parties, and busloads of Gaelic football fans – their loud laughter and boisterous energy filling the shop.

But just as laughter filled the off-licence, so did sorrow. Some customers arrived alone, offering smiles and jokes with a sadness behind their eyes that I couldn't unsee. Others didn't bother to hide their despair. Heavy sighs. Quiet words. Invisible weight.

Immersed in the full spectrum of human emotion, I came to love the job. It was humbling. Looking back, I can see a parallel between what I witnessed behind that counter and what therapists see in snapshots of people's lives. I've heard hairdressers and barbers say the same.

While I enjoyed these jobs, I never saw them as my end goal. I wanted a career that would break past the barriers my parents had faced. They had been denied opportunities, and I was determined to take mine. I wanted to use both education and work to avoid the financial hardship they endured. I was ready to break the cycle and build a future.

So you can imagine my overwhelming joy when I achieved two A's and a B in my A-levels – in physics, biology, and chemistry – and was offered a place at Queen's University Belfast. I couldn't wait to discover my adult self.

I began my Master of Pharmacy degree at Queen's. There, I met some unforgettable people in the halls – Colleen from Keady, a musical fella from Derry, a banter king from Banbridge, and a traditional musician from Donegal.

Everything was looking up. Life was blossoming as it should.

But I didn't know that my emerging self wouldn't have a chance.

She was about to die.

The Flood, Spring 2006:
Fresher Year

"After a traumatic experience, the human system of self-preservation seems to go onto permanent alert, as if the danger might return at any moment."

— Judith Lewis Herman

Chapter 7: When Everything Changed

Get free.
Struggle.
Body acts out – no.
No, I say.

A sharp rise in fear.
His piercing, evil stare
tells me all I need to know:
No chance.

My body falls limp,
refusing my brain's command.
Terror.
No chance of survival.

I'm going to die.

Feel tears roll
down my right cheek.
The switch is flicked.
Life ending.
Life ended.

Nothingness.
In and out of nothingness.
Feel the tears.
Feel him.
It's over.

Awake now.
Body here.

Body numb.
He asks if I'm okay.
I do not know why he asks.
I do not understand anything.

Self is gone.
She is gone.
I am gone.

Call my friend.
You must have asked for it
the friend implies.

I must have asked for it.
It repeats,
over and over,
in the space between my ears.

Must carry on.
The mask goes on.
I watch her
go through the motions.
Shows up, ticks boxes.
Her body moves on –
she does not.

But she doesn't know it. Not yet.

***

It's difficult to put my experience into words.

There are moments in life when language fails – and even the poem above doesn't come close to capturing what happened to me.

In that moment, when I was completely overpowered, my body and brain registered it as a threat to life. But what I experienced wasn't just life-threatening. My response was primal, rooted in survival. There was no logic, no reasoning. Only sensation. Only instinct. Time became irrelevant. Shock stretched far beyond the moment itself. **Nothing made sense.**

And that not-making-sense stayed with me for a very long time.

Chapter 8: A&E, May 2006

I'm sitting on what feels like a hard plastic chair.
There are people all around me – **too many**.
Bodies moving in every direction.
The lights are harsh.
Too harsh.
It's too bright.
Too noisy.
Too many sounds.
Too many smells.

My heart is pounding.
I want out of here.

"Come with me," a voice says, appearing from nowhere.
Automatically, I stand and follow.

I'm taken to a small corner.
I can still hear the voices – loud and overlapping.
The lights are still piercing.
I hear the wavering hum of electricity as they flicker.
I wish someone would turn them off.

A woman – maybe a nurse, maybe a doctor, I cannot tell – pulls
the thin hospital curtain around us.
Only partway.
It doesn't block the noise.
It doesn't block the light.
It doesn't feel private.

People walking past can still look in.
I try to make eye contact with her.

I focus, really hard.

She speaks in a clipped, clinical tone.
"So, you requested the morning-after pill?"

"Yes," I say, just as automatically as I moved from the chair.

I'm frightened.
I'm confused.
I don't know how I got here.

Please help.

But I don't have words.
No words.
They won't come.
Where are my words?

I keep staring into her eyes, trying to talk with mine.
Why can't she see how scared I am?
Why can't she hear me?

"Was it consensual?" she asks.

The word lands from a distance.
It echoes.
Consensual?

But I don't register that she's speaking to me.
Nothing makes sense.

She continues.
"Do you have any bruises?"
Oh. She's talking to me.

But I'm still confused.
Her questions come too fast.
Too sharp.

Is this real?

I stay silent.

Bruises.
Bruises.
Bruises.

If I had bruises, I'd feel them, wouldn't I?

"No bruises," I say.

Why did she ask that?
I just want the pill.

This is so confusing.

"So you have no bruises," she says again, her voice a little firmer.
"But can you tell me if it was consensual sex?"

Consensual.

That word again.

Is this a real conversation?

It's hard to look her in the eye now.
I look down.
The floor is easier.

I hyperfocus.
Block everything else out – the noise, the light, the smells.
The floor becomes my anchor.

Consent.
Consensual.
Consent.
The words circle in my head.

Isn't all sex consensual?

Then: the short skirt.
The drink.
The short skirt.

The drink.
Over and over.

There's not enough air in this room.

"Anna, did you consent to sex?"

Her voice cuts through again.
I glance at the gap in the curtain.

I need to get out of here.

I must have asked for it, I think.
My friend says I asked for it.
The short skirt.
The drink.

I nod. Just slightly.
No words come out.

"Okay. Consensual," she says, moving on.
"When was your last period?"

I stare at her mouth now.
It's easier than looking in her eyes.

My period?
I don't know.

Everything's blurring – noise, light, smell.
Her mouth moves in slow motion,
but the words come too fast.

I know I have to say something if I want to leave.

"Last week," I whisper.

She keeps talking – pregnancy, chances, statistics.
It's too much.
I just want the pill.

She says something about blood pressure,
then wraps a cuff around my arm.

I watch her do it, detached.
Like it's happening to someone else.

But when she says she's going to the pharmacy to get the pill,
I feel the faintest drop of relief.

I return to the floor.
I wait.

And wait.

And wait.

It feels like a long time now.

She returns.
More words.

I stare at her lips.
They move,
but I cannot hear anything.

Then I'm handed a packet.
I'm discharged.

I walk back to my halls
without realising I'm walking.

Suddenly, I'm sitting on my bed.

I want a shower.
A second shower.
I feel dirty.
I need to wash again.

I take a shower.

Then I sit on a towel at the edge of my bed, naked, and see the bruises.

I remember the nurse asking me about bruises.
Now I see them.

Huge, dark bruises
along the inside of my thighs.

But they do not look like my legs.
They cannot be mine.

Time passes.
I don't remember showering.

Then I touch my hair.
It's slightly damp.
I don't remember washing it.
I think the shower cap must have leaked.

I don't know how long I've been sitting here.

Then – my phone pings.
I flinch.

A text from *him*.

He asks if I'm okay.
He says he wants to meet.

I don't understand
why he's asking if I'm okay.

He asked me that this morning.

I get dressed.
I text him back.
I tell him where I am.

Shattered

"There are wounds that never show on the body that are deeper and more hurtful than anything that bleeds."

— LAURELL K. HAMILTON

Chapter 9: In Search of Myself

Psychoanalysis triggered a long trip down memory lane. Most of my analytical work happened in between sessions. Marek and my son were incredibly patient with me as I moved through this process. While Marek entertained our child, I spent many evenings frantically searching for information.

I'd find myself rummaging through my dad's dark and dusty attic, the smell of old paper and forgotten years hanging in the air. I dug through piles of paperwork, mined my email archives, and flicked through aged photo albums with an almost desperate energy. I was looking for something, though I didn't know what. Maybe I was searching for evidence of my "self", the self I had lost *that night*.

One afternoon, I asked Marek to share with me some emails he'd exchanged with my mum – messages about concerns for my mental health during the early years of our relationship. Reading through them, I was overwhelmed by a wave of nausea. In an instant, I was transported back. I could smell the air from those years, thick with confusion, uncertainty, and a deep sense of being lost.

Those emails revealed what I hadn't known then: even though the political troubles had long subsided, and the British chopper base had been decommissioned in Flagstaff, a different kind of trouble was brewing inside our home in Newry. Quietly, a family inquisition had formed around me.

Unbeknownst to me, messages were being exchanged. My mum took the lead, lovingly reaching out to Marek, my then-boyfriend, in an effort to understand what was happening to me. But it was an impossible task. I couldn't explain it – because I didn't understand it myself.

It wasn't until I began my own internal inquisition, through psychoanalysis, that I started to uncover the truth of what was happening to me back then.

Sadly, I cannot turn back time to provide my mum with the answers she so desperately sought. My family, like most families, moved on with their own lives. They may not even remember the inquisition as they have had their own trials and tribulations since then. For them, perhaps, it's all a distant memory, if remembered at all.

But for me, as I sift through old photos and messages, it's as though it happened only yesterday.

I wish I could respond to my mum's emails. I wish I could tell her my story. But she is no longer here.

What I can do now is share it with you.

Chapter 10: What the Picture Didn't Show

One particular photo, taken in the earlier years following the rape, gives me the chills because I barely recognise myself. My tiny frame is defined by my skeletal structure, with little muscle or fat to cushion it. While the correct label, *anorexic*, was never applied, it had started to become obvious that I was significantly scrawnier than I had been before. I recall Toodles telling me that her friends had expressed concern about the weight I had lost in such a short time.

What others observed was nothing compared to how I felt – or didn't feel.

Around this time, I remember being in a physiology lab at university, draped in a white coat that barely masked my deprived body. While the coat hid my bony frame, I felt weak, almost faint, and exposed, as though the fabric couldn't conceal the emptiness within. My anxiety was palpable, forcing me into awareness of my physical symptoms. I knew something was broken inside me, but I didn't know how to ask for help.

I felt exhausted and kept glancing at the clock, desperate for the class to end.

The professor called for a volunteer to demonstrate a blood sugar test. He was met with silence and blank stares; though he wasn't in a rush, as he continued preparing a few other tests. However, it was all too quiet for me, and the anxiety was rising further into my chest. I thought, *What the heck, let's just get this class over with*. Besides, there was a quiet curiosity within me to see what my sugar levels actually were, given that I hadn't been nourishing myself properly. And for a fleeting moment, I thought that if I were met with a low blood sugar result, someone might see me, truly see that I needed help.

The tutor pricked my finger, and on reading the result, he said, "You need to eat something." I forced a brief smile, and without further comment, we continued on with the lesson.

Reflecting on this memory, I realise that a lot was happening during that time. I made certain changes that I had rationalised in my mind. One of the most impulsive changes was quitting my job at the off-licence. I rang my manager and used the excuse that my shifts no longer worked with my university schedule, which was partly true, but it wasn't the main reason for leaving.

The slight tone of disappointment in his voice echoed between my ears. Looking back, I imagine he felt let down. After working there for nearly two years, it wasn't the best way to quit. I should have done the decent thing and spoken to him face to face. But I didn't understand myself what was going on with me. Hiding was just easier than facing anyone.

Despite the unacknowledged feelings, life continued as I thought it should. I moved through the motions of daily, weekly, and monthly life, adapting myself to whatever was expected of me. I perfected the mask I wore – the smile on my face – until it became second nature. I almost believed I had become the mask itself. I developed habits, obsessions, and avoidance strategies that I thought were necessary for my survival.

Little did I know that while I could hide from my own pain, the trauma would never leave me. Without treatment, my wound would endure – constantly insulted, both in the workplace and at home – festering and growing, until it finally demanded my attention.

Chapter 11: Circling the Wound

The first lesson I learned in therapy was that a skilled therapist can hear what you're not saying – the spaces between your words, the silence hidden in your voice, and what your body is trying to tell them. David read me from our very first meeting, and as our sessions continued, his ability somewhat irritated me. But since this was the service I was seeking, I couldn't exactly complain. With his sharp observational skills and subtle guidance, the truth-unravelling process began quickly. Within just a few sessions, I had already confronted that night.

***

"Anna, I've noticed some signs that are often associated with trauma," David says gently, "and I do not think they're entirely related to your mother's passing. I'm wondering about your past experiences – if anything might have happened earlier in your life that felt out of your control or extremely difficult."

I sit awkwardly across from him and glance towards the window, unsure where else to look. I don't know what to say, and we fall into another silence. But this one doesn't bother me. The noise in my head – a tangled swirl of thoughts – is loud enough to distract me from the weirdness of having these kinds of conversations with a stranger.

One thought, more persistent than the rest, nags at me: What is he expecting me to say?

Time passes, I think, but I've no idea how much. Just as I realise it's probably my turn to speak, David breaks the silence.

"What are you thinking?"

"I'm not really sure, ehm…" I start.

"Go on," he encourages, his tone calm and steady.

With a few more ums and pauses, I speak, mostly to fill the space. I feel silly, like what I'm saying isn't really that important.

"I remember something… during my first year at university, but ehm…"

David nods, inviting me to continue.

"I, ehm, woke up to a man…" I begin, then tell him, haltingly, about a night out in Newry that ended at a house party. I woke up to someone inside me. I do not go into detail, but I say enough.

I stop, and there's a pause.

David repeats my words back to me gently, without changing them. Then he adds, "Anna, we have about fifteen minutes left today. What you've just shared sounds very serious. And what you've described… many would understand that as rape."

I hear him, but the word doesn't land. It floats somewhere outside me, like it was meant for someone else. I don't know what to think. It can't be rape, can it?

Instead, my mind jumps to something more urgent: I need to remember to get my son ready for nursery. And that reminds me, I had a really difficult morning with him. That's something I actually need to talk about.

***

When I first disclosed the sexual violation I experienced in 2006, I avoided accessing all of my memories of the event. While those memories were always there, buried somewhere in my mind, I had chosen to shut them away. I never wanted to open that box, and I avoided it for a long time.

Many sessions went by where I had everything else to talk about – bar the rape. And in the early phases of therapy, even when I did bring it up, I didn't speak of it in any real detail. It just didn't seem that important. I didn't realise then that facing the truth was so difficult that my mind had started trivialising it. Ideas, distractions, and rationalisations were some of the ways I tried to avoid it.

I had always thought rape was something that happened to other people, something you read about in the news. Surely, it didn't happen to me. And even if it did, was it really such a big deal? It was a physical attack, and it was a long time ago – ancient history. I told myself I was over it. But once I acknowledged that what I experienced was rape, I had to work through intense feelings of self-blame. The phrase "I must have asked for it" crept back in, quietly and cruelly. I worked through these feelings and memories intermittently between analysing the weeks, months and years after the rape.

When it finally came time to verbalise my memories in more detail, I had already emotionally detached from the experience. That detachment made it easier to speak about, just as it's made it possible for me to write this now. Without that distance, I don't think I could recount my story at all.

Chapter 12: The Comfort That Wasn't

For a brief period, following the rape, I relied on heavy drinking, masking my need for alcohol under the guise of student-style partying. During that time, alcohol abuse and wild nights became my coping mechanisms. But eventually, I turned inward, cutting out my social circle and retreating from nightlife altogether.

I was unaware that I was suffering from post-traumatic stress disorder (PTSD). I was also unaware that I was autistic, and that the PTSD was compounding my autistic traits, and vice versa. Being unaware didn't mean that my PTSD and autistic needs didn't need to be met. At my most vulnerable state, those needs became crucial. I yearned for routine, predictability, familiarity, and above all, security. I needed safety, so I clung to those closest to me.

At the time, I saw *my friend*, someone I had known for years, as one of my biggest lifelines. I had followed them closely for years, like a shadow following a moving figure, always believing they were my safe place. We shared moments I thought were meaningful – until I started to question whether we valued them in the same way. This non-conformist friend was the type to shock me into belly-rolling laughter with their theatrical stories and deliberate outrageousness. To me, they were like a peacock in a room full of pigeons. Even though they seemed more mature and sensible around others, I paid no heed to the different faces they showed. At the time, I believed I was the person they trusted most. Whether that was true or just what I needed to believe, I'll never know. Unaware of my own needs and boundaries at the time, I often let the gravitational pull of others shape my direction. When that familiar connection faded, I couldn't stay. Belfast felt too exposed, too stark. I left, even though I was still in the middle of my degree – not because I had a plan, but because staying felt unbearable.

I craved familiarity and sought protection in those I knew, unaware that I wasn't always great at seeking safety in the right places. My strong attachment style hindered my ability to spot danger, even when the signs were glaring. And looking back, I wonder if some people sensed it.

Masking And Minimising

"We are taught to smile, even when we are breaking. To shrink, so others can breathe more easily."

— NIKITA GILL

Chapter 13: Called It Stress

Apart from the weeks immediately following the rape, there were no obvious outward signs of trauma – at least not right away. But months later, things began to change. I developed a deep apathy and disinterest in my studies and student life. The motivation and drive I once had to succeed in my career disappeared during my second year at university. By my third year, my lecture attendance was dropping quickly, and commuting to university became increasingly difficult.

I had been travelling daily on the Rooney's bus, which still runs from Newry to Queen's. But panic and anxiety started to disrupt that routine. I started experiencing panic episodes on the bus, and one day I asked to get off before it had even departed for Belfast.

I decided to visit my GP. I didn't know what was wrong with me. I only knew that I was experiencing overwhelming somatic feelings that had suddenly intensified that day. I hadn't connected the dots. I hadn't linked the rape to the panic. How could I? Thinking about the rape wasn't something I allowed myself to do.

Time was marching on, and my unprocessed trauma was quietly compounding. The longer it went unspoken, the harder it became to understand what was happening to me.

With little to go on, my GP inferred that my symptoms of panic "must be related to your studies", and prescribed antidepressants and anxiolytics and recommended self-help books. The once capable girl I had been – the focused, driven young woman – was now struggling. And as the words "it must be your studies" echoed in my mind, I started to believe them. It seemed to make sense at the time, so I followed that narrative.

I was diagnosed with general anxiety disorder (GAD), and that label stuck. With a quick diagnosis and an even quicker prescription, I was put on medication that, in some ways, only further numbed me from the trauma I hadn't yet faced. I don't remember if I was offered a referral to mental health services, and if I was, the importance of therapy was never stressed. After all, as the GP said, the problem was probably just academic stress and dealing with that was the objective. And so, I took the tablets and just got on with it.

Chapter 14: Playing the Survivor

"Survival is not about being fearless. It's about making a decision, getting on and doing it."

— BEAR GRYLLS

Unaware that I had lost trust in everyone – including my GPs – I carried on with life the only way I knew how. I clung to the safety of familiar "social rules and constructs" I had learned to believe in. As an autistic person – though I didn't know it yet – I had always navigated the world through learned patterns and rules.

Familiarity – whether in people, places or routines – offered me a sense of safety. I trusted my GPs, believing the health system existed to care for its patients. I trusted my friend, because I believed friends were meant to care for one another. I trusted my family, assuming they knew me inside and out and had my best interests at heart.

While most of their intentions were likely good, things didn't always turn out the way I expected. The rules I had lived by – the social scripts I relied on – were just that: learned. But they did not yield the anticipated outcomes. A sense of safety doesn't always equal actual safety, and I didn't know that yet.

Coming to understand that I had no real agency – that deep, internal belief in one's ability to manage one's own life – was a hard pill to swallow. I was swept up by my wounds and more vulnerable because of them.

The only thing I knew for certain was that I had to survive. And seeking comfort in the familiar was the only survival strategy I had.

Chapter 15: Triggers

Through my work with my therapist, I began to see the connections in the puzzle pieces. The version of myself I had created – both for others and for me – was not the true picture. The truth was hidden beneath layers of trauma.

I came to realise that on the day, down to the very hour, that someone brutally stole my freedom, a part of me froze in time. Outwardly, I appeared to move on, but inside, I remained stuck. Life around me pressed forward; I went through the motions, but I wasn't truly part of it. While my peers progressed, I stayed behind, unknowingly tethered to the past.

No matter how far I tried to run from the trauma, it clung to me, shaping every part of my world. Just like that time I had to get off my usual bus journey to university, gripped by panic. What I didn't understand then was that the reaction came from somatic memory – trauma stored in the body – from that very lonely journey I had made to Belfast just hours after the rape. The smell of the bus, the hum of the engine, the feel of the seat beneath me – each of these sensory details transported me back to that moment, triggering fear and distress.

Understanding that events, places, smells, sounds – even the tiniest sensations – could ignite trauma responses was another turning point. For years, I had believed I was simply "prone to anxiety", as one GP had suggested. But something deeper, more specific, was going on. And I had only just begun to uncover it.

It was in 2021, fifteen years later, that I finally grasped a life-changing truth: these experiences, these symptoms, were not *me*. I didn't have to be defined by them anymore. I didn't have to berate myself for not doing things as easily as others did. I didn't have to punish myself for needing more time, more rest, more gentleness.

Becoming aware of this truth was one thing. Believing it – really *believing* it – and releasing the deep-seated self-blame was something else. Could I really separate myself from my symptoms? Could I dig beneath the layers of trauma and find the real me waiting there? Or would I drown in grief for all the years lost – years when trauma muted my voice, clouded my joy, and shaped an identity that was never truly mine?

So many paths lay before me, each one demanding exploration. Do I begin by processing the event itself? Do I grieve the person I might have been? Or do I nurture the person I still might become?

There were no easy answers. Only puzzle pieces, scattered across the table of my life. And at last, I had begun to pick them up.

The road to healing stretched long before me, and with cautious hope, I had just taken my first steps.

Chapter 16: Something I Ate

I enter the session completely exhausted. There's no energy left for small talk or beating around the bush, so I go straight in.

"David, last night I had one of those episodes again, you know, the ones I get at night. I've had them for years. All I feel is panic, racing heart, sweating... ehm... feeling really afraid." I can't remember if I've told him about these episodes before, but I speak as if I have. It feels like something he should already know.

He looks at me with quiet concern and asks, "Can you tell me more about what happened?"

I slump further into the chair. I don't want to explain. I don't want to be here, talking about this. But I take a sharp breath and start. The words come out in a rush, almost automatically. I recount the panic, the chest-tightening, the dread that doesn't have a name, the endless trips to the bathroom. I finish with: "Like always, the vomiting is the only thing that brings relief. I think it was around 4 a.m. when I finally settled."

There's a pause. Then David speaks, gently but deliberately. "You said these episodes happen often. Have you been to your GPs about them?"

I take another sharp breath. I feel a flicker of frustration. I do not want to be redirected to my doctors again – I've phoned them several times over the years about this.

"Yes, on different occasions," I reply. "Once they told me it was likely something I ate. Another time, they said it was probably IBS. One said it was 'just one of those things'. Even when I called out-of-hours during one of the episodes, they told me it was most likely a COVID fever and that I should isolate; they thought my internal shaking was a sign that I had a fever. I don't call the doctors anymore. They don't know what it is."

David watches me with deepening concern. "Do you remember when they first began?"

I think for a moment.

"I remember the first full episode. I'd had an Indian takeaway that night. I thought it was food poisoning at the time... but it's happened so many times since. It can't just be something I ate."

He leans in slightly, not physically, but with presence.

"When was that?"

I hesitate, searching.

"Ehm... I think it was autumn 2006. Yes, definitely. It was one of the first takeaways I had in Ireland with Marek. We'd just started seeing each other."

Another pause. Then David asks, with the calm precision that marks his more pointed questions: "Anna, what year was it that you were raped?" There's no tension in his tone, but something shifts in the room.

I answer quietly. "2006."

I really don't know what that's got to do with my vomiting episodes. I go home, not quite understanding the session, but something inside me knows.

***

Diagnosis And Realisation

Chapter 17: Called by Its Name

Uncovering the root cause of my symptoms led me to seek formal confirmation of my diagnosis. I didn't want my distress to be continually misinterpreted as something that it wasn't. I needed clarity. I needed truth. And I needed that truth to be acknowledged, not hidden behind the obscurity of an anxiety disorder label. So I arranged to see a psychiatrist, who confirmed that I did, in fact, have PTSD. He also suggested that I report the rape to the police. After hearing my story and reviewing my medical history, he said there was more than enough clinical evidence to support my case. At that stage, I hadn't seriously considered going to the police, but the idea had now been planted.

In 2023, I received the written confirmation of my PTSD diagnosis. Seeing it in black and white – my name alongside the words "Post-Traumatic Stress Disorder" – brought a visceral reaction. The gravity of it all suddenly hit me. It was real. The fog of dissociation that had hung over the memory of the rape began to lift. This was no longer something tucked away in a dusty corner of my mind; it was now part of my medical record. My life.

Although I was still unaware of my autism during that phase of therapy, my autistic traits – like my need for clarity, structure, and understanding – compelled me to dig deeper. I felt uneasy about how swiftly I'd been diagnosed with GAD and depression by my GPs years earlier. As a pharmacist, I've always taken a serious interest in the effective treatment of health conditions, and this was no exception. The more I examined my own medical records, the more irritated I became. I found careless phrases like "patient prone to anxiety" scattered throughout. I realised how a single vague note had been lazily recycled at different points in my file. It felt like no one had truly tried to understand me, just quick judgments and even quicker prescriptions. How many more of us, I wondered, are mislabelled and medicated into silence?

Learning about the full spectrum of PTSD symptoms – flashbacks, hypervigilance, panic, dissociation, numbing – was illuminating. I saw myself in every description. I realised how deeply embedded these symptoms were in my day-to-day life. And with that realisation came a wave of frustration. Why didn't anyone see this? How could the people closest to me – doctors, professors, colleagues, friends, family – not recognise what I was going through? Why didn't they ask the right questions?

The only person who truly saw me was David; that's what he was trained to do. For everyone else I had interacted with over the years, it was as if my trauma had been invisible, even though the symptoms were written all over me. But they, like I once had, must have assumed that my struggles were simply part of my personality: that I was just sensitive, just anxious, just moody. I felt an unfamiliar surge of anger, something I had rarely allowed myself to feel. But David had sensed it long before I did. I was always a few steps behind him when it came to learning about myself.

Eventually, I accepted what my clenched fists were trying to tell me. I had to find out where that anger was coming from. Where had the support been when I needed it most? Why had it been absent? If my PTSD had been recognised and addressed closer to the time of the rape, maybe it wouldn't have become so severe. I needed to understand why I had gone unnoticed for so long, and what that revealed not just about the systems around me, but also about the silence I had been forced to endure.

Chapter 18: Lost in Plain Sight

"The greatest thing in the world is to know how to belong to oneself."

— MICHEL DE MONTAIGNE

To understand why I went unnoticed for seventeen years, I had to examine my behaviour and circumstances from 2006 to the present day. After years of therapy and reflection, I realised that my invisibility wasn't the result of a single reason, but many. My trauma response, the normalisation of trauma symptoms – by me and by others – the masking of my symptoms, the shame I carried, the cultural push for toxic positivity, the busyness of life, and failures in our healthcare system all played a role.

One of the biggest reasons I remained unseen was trauma itself. PTSD made it extremely difficult – often impossible – for me to understand, process, or verbalise what *had happened* to me and what *was happening* to me. This PTSD barrier was complex and perhaps rooted in a childhood trauma I only began to uncover in the later stages of therapy.

It was also during this time that I learned of my autism diagnosis. Much like politics and religion are entangled in Northern Ireland, often fuelling unrest, my autism and PTSD were deeply entangled, creating an internal conflict of their own. Both my childhood trauma and my autism are topics I've only just begun to process in 2024, and they're too complex to fully elaborate on yet.

Navigating life meant constantly oscillating between fight, flight, freeze, friend, and flop – the five Fs – with only fleeting periods of "normal" in between. Life after rape was nothing like life before. I developed new difficulties and disabilities, and found everyday challenges harder than ever. The struggles linked to my autism worsened significantly. Simple tasks – going to the supermarket, driving, meeting friends, handling work – became overwhelming, and sometimes impossible. What others took for granted felt out of reach for me.

What's worse, I didn't understand *why*. With no obvious explanation for my symptoms, disabilities, inabilities or struggles, I blamed myself. I convinced myself I could not "do life" like my peers. And as my self-confidence in every area of my life eroded, I became better at masking it, concealing my struggles, because I was ashamed of them, ashamed of myself.

The fatigue was constant. Pretending I was "okay" drained me. I began shutting myself off from opportunities, big and small. The vomiting episodes became routine; I dismissed them as "just one of those things". A GP had once said as much, and I clung to that explanation. It took therapy to uncover that these were panic attacks directly linked to the rape. I invalidated every sign and symptom of my trauma – and in doing so, I invalidated myself.

As this "new" and wounded person, I had relegated myself to the lowest rung of the ladder, though outwardly, I didn't always appear that way. I became increasingly vulnerable to further abuse. My ability to advocate for myself vanished. As a result, a destructive spiral was set in motion, worsening with each blow. I never saw myself as vulnerable, but now I face this reality head-on. Yet to those close to me, I was known only through the mask I wore. As I minimised my symptoms, so did they.

Cultural factors – toxic positivity and the overwhelming busyness of life – also prevented my "scream" from being heard. My emotional reactions to seemingly minor events, a product of emotional dysregulation, were often met with minimising responses or toxic positivity, making it nearly impossible to uncover the root cause. Society expects us all to thrive, not just survive. The illusion that everything is within reach for everyone else made it even harder for me to recognise or acknowledge my own suffering. While others appeared to thrive, I was barely holding on. And so I kept up appearances. I kept the mask on.

And when we're all consumed by the busyness of our own lives, caught up in our own experiences, it becomes hard to see when someone else is drowning. I was no exception. My trauma went unseen, and I likely missed the signs in others too. That affected my relationships in ways I'm still trying to understand.

And, of course, I was also failed by the healthcare system. No professional I saw – including the one I consulted just hours after the attack – recognised my trauma or responded to the red flags. My cries for help went unheard. The lack of trauma-informed care is deplorable. In a society where trauma is so widespread, it's not unreasonable to expect our primary healthcare providers to be trained to recognise it.

The longer the delay in diagnosis, the more difficult the healing process becomes. I believe if my autism had been identified in childhood, my vulnerabilities could have been spotted much sooner. And maybe I wouldn't have appeared so vulnerable to the predator who singled me out in a room full of neurotypical women.

Unveiling the disconnect between my inner world and how the world saw me forced me to revisit the life that unfolded in the years after the rape.

Exile and Adaptation

Surviving Abroad

Chapter 19: Crossing Borders to Survive

It was 2010, four and a half years after the attack, and I had just completed my pre-registration pharmacist training – a year of professional training and practice following my master's degree in pharmacy. Considering everything I had been through and was still going through, it felt like nothing short of a miracle that I had managed to finish my degree and my registration year with the Pharmaceutical Society of Northern Ireland.

But because my trauma and autism remained undiagnosed, no reasonable accommodations were made. I didn't know the playing field wasn't level. I was a neurodivergent, traumatised young woman, exerting extraordinary effort to achieve the same goals as my neurotypical peers. I didn't see that at the time. Instead, I blamed myself for my fatigue and struggles. I left no room for compassion for myself. Only in 2024 would I begin to understand the true weight I'd been carrying.

Looking back, it's no surprise I found myself unemployed – a newly qualified pharmacist battling imposter syndrome, fearful of socialising, and paralysed by a terror of driving that I couldn't explain. I was done with Ireland. Done with the UK. To say I was discontent would be an understatement. I needed to escape. I searched for opportunities abroad, driven by that familiar urge to run. I had discovered that not only was I unhappy at home, but I no longer felt safe there. I was stuck between a rock and a hard place.

Then I found it: a pre-Brexit, fully funded European Union programme – the Leonardo da Vinci Programme – offering recent graduates an opportunity to live and work abroad. Open to all in Northern Ireland, both "orange" and "green", it felt like my ticket to freedom. I convinced myself this was the key to my career development, the edge my CV needed. But beneath that rationalisation, I knew I was chasing something deeper: a promise of a new life. I applied. I was accepted.

With a painted-on smile and the occasional social media post, I quietly slipped out of the country. No farewell drinks, no good-byes. I didn't believe I deserved them. Having abandoned university life midway through my degree, I'd missed out on forging lasting friendships and the full university experience. Of the few friends I had, I feared no one would bother to show up.

I left behind Marek, who had, ironically, only recently moved to Ireland to be with me. I felt emotional about leaving him. I couldn't imagine life without him, but part of me had to run, not from him, from myself. I convinced myself that this was the break I needed. I told myself that the *dolce vita* was waiting for me, that I would find peace once I landed in Florence. My head was filled with romantic notions of Italy, shaped by books and movies like *Under the Tuscan Sun*. I spent the weeks before I left listening endlessly to Italian pop and opera. Ligabue. Andrea Bocelli. I imagined living out the best parts of those stories.

But the *dolce vita* I had envisioned turned out to be far from the life that awaited me.

Chapter 20: Behind the Aperitivo Smile

In Italy, I shared snippets of my story on social media – a glimpse into the internal battle I was fighting. But those glimpses barely scratched the surface. I framed my inner turmoil as an "Ireland versus Italy" struggle, but the real conflict was between me and myself.

What happened in Florence was both beautiful and brutal. The beautiful moments – the ones I'm happy to share – fit neatly into the clichés of *la dolce vita*: the wine, the sun, the Italians, and, of course, the food. The warmth of the Tuscan sun that kissed my skin, the intoxicating scent of espresso drifting through narrow streets, the chatter and laughter spilling from cafés – it all painted a picture of romance and indulgence.

I immediately bonded with a local woman named Giulia Evangelisti. We met at a small pizzeria called Gustapizza on Via Maggio. Our friendship blossomed, and soon I was welcomed into her family: her father Claudio (now sadly passed away), her mother Sandra, and her brother Niccolò.

Claudio cooked for me often. Evenings with them were filled with the smells of home-cooked meals and the smoothness of Italian wine slipping down my throat. The wine gave me just enough courage to speak Italian more freely. The Evangelistis' home became a safe haven for me. Their warmth and hospitality helped me feel a sense of normalcy and alleviated some of the isolation I felt. They offered me safety without even knowing it, and that kindness will stay with me forever.

Then there was Mauretta Bernardini, a local Florentine, and her husband Geoff, an English *straniero* (foreigner). They were my neighbours, and they came to my rescue the day my apartment was ransacked.

I came home from my placement to find my belongings – even my underwear – strewn across the floor and bed. The air felt heavy with violation. I was too afraid to stay alone that night, so Mauretta and Geoff took me in, like I was their daughter. We didn't realise at the time, but the violation of my personal space had triggered a retraumatisation. By offering me shelter, they offered me safety, and I will never forget their kindness.

I also lived with two sets of young Spanish women. I could write a book about the "craic" we shared. They spoke no English; I spoke no Spanish. We communicated in a delightful mix of *Spanglish*, *Itanglish*, and *Spallion* – gestures and charades filling the gaps. Our loud, spontaneous, uncontrollable laughter became a soundtrack to our days – a kind of therapy. One of them, Apolonia Domínguez Fernández – Polly – from Andalusia, became a dear friend. Together, we took buses to random Tuscan villages, dined, drank, and shared hours in each other's company. It's astonishing how two people who didn't share a common language could connect so deeply.

Polly filled our apartment with joy – flamenco dancing as she cooked Spanish omelettes, cheering me up with her infectious energy and her signature greeting: "*Ana, Ana, che pasa?*" Even on my worst days, she reminded me why life was worth living.

But there was a darker side to Florence. After my assault, I struggled to establish boundaries. As an unhealed autistic rape victim, I didn't even know what healthy boundaries looked like. Moving to a foreign country, where I didn't speak the language and had no tools to protect myself, was overwhelming. In hindsight, it was like being thrown to the lions.

*** ***

In the middle of the session, something clicks – a sudden, searing realisation of just how exposed and vulnerable I've been. It lands in my chest like a punch. The pain is so sharp, so absurd, that I erupt into uncontrollable laughter, bubbling up from somewhere dark and wild. It's not funny, not even close. But it's as if my body doesn't know where else to put the pain.

David watches me gently, his eyes soft but alert. "Why are you laughing?" he asks, his voice low, careful.

When the laughter finally dies down, leaving behind a hollow ache in my throat, I manage a weak smile. "You either laugh or cry."

***

The harsh reality of Florence is that I fell back into daily drinking. The wine slipped down too easily, numbing the overwhelming emotions clawing their way to the surface. I slid back into a state of worthlessness – the same despair I'd felt after the assault in 2006. Vulnerable, unprotected, I became a target for those who were savvy at spotting and exploiting that vulnerability. By the time my placement ended, I felt numb. Disconnected from myself, from everyone – even Marek, the man I had promised to marry before leaving for Italy. When I returned to Ireland, I felt like I'd left a part of myself behind in Florence. I convinced myself that my life was there, and I began planning my return.

Landing in Ireland felt like the end of the world. I was back to square one – worse off than before. The illusion of *la dolce vita* kept calling me back. I was ready to abandon everything: my relationships, my job search, my career.

My apathy was evident to everyone around me, especially my mother and Marek. I ended my relationship with Marek, calling for a "break". My family saw the change. The whispers began – born of concern, but painful all the same. They couldn't possibly understand what I was going through. How could they? I didn't understand it myself.

There were moments when the despair was so deep I would retreat to my room, lie on my bed, and cry for hours. My mother, already struggling with depression, didn't know how to cope with my turmoil. Our simultaneous mental health struggles fed into each other, deepening the spiral. I remember a call from Toodles in Australia, sharing her concern about Mum, saying Mum felt she had lost me. Little did they know how truly lost I was, and yet I was unable to verbally communicate what I was going through.

Toodles was far away, Cuddles was busy with university, and Mum was feeling low herself. We both needed support, we were both struggling, so I dried my tears.

Losing Worth

Chapter 21: Same Feeling, Different Room

I went to my NHS GP with an incidental finding of an ovarian cyst that I'd learned about in Italy. Before I knew it, I was scheduled for surgery just a few days after my 25th birthday. I arrived at the hospital, anxious and sleep-deprived. My mum accompanied me, sitting by my side as I waited in the ward. The staff prepped me for surgery, but provided no information about the schedule, the surgeon, or the procedure itself. I could barely speak to my mum, but her presence was the one thing grounding me.

Despite being a qualified pharmacist, I felt like a child, completely at the mercy of others. A student surgeon visited shortly before the surgery. He was calm and professional, but I remember how unsettled I felt. He looked so much like the man who assaulted me in 2006. The resemblance was uncanny, triggering something I wouldn't fully understand until much later.

He explained the plan was for keyhole surgery, but it might switch to open surgery at any point. There was a risk of losing my ovary. I didn't feel much about that – my anxiety was more centred on the procedure itself, the anaesthesia, the uncertainty. I asked for an anxiolytic to calm my nerves, but he refused, worried it might interfere with the anaesthesia. He left, and I still had no idea when the surgery would happen.

Without warning, two nurses appeared, brisk and business like. They wheeled me towards the operating theatre. That's when the tears came. As the elevator doors closed, one muttered to the other, speaking as if I wasn't even there: "Mr *** *(surgeon)* won't put up with that."

At that moment, I knew I wasn't supposed to react or flinch. If I did, Mr *** wouldn't be pleased.

On entering the theatre, I was surrounded by a flurry of activity – surgeon, anaesthetist, nurses, all doing their checks, laying out tubes, needles, tools, and medications. It felt impersonal, like I was a car at the mechanic's, getting its parts fixed. The anaesthetist checked my blood pressure and heart rate, and it was only then that he noticed I was having an anxiety attack. Reflecting on this, it's almost tragic that a medical practitioner could only detect a mental health episode by measuring blood pressure.

No one had thought to ask how I was feeling.

"You need to calm down, or this surgery cannot proceed," the anaesthetist warned. "I can't administer anaesthesia if your blood pressure is this high."

I asked the surgeon, "How long will I be under?"

"That's none of your concern," he replied.

The last thing I remember is their discussion about my high blood pressure and heart rate, and then the surgeon, clipped and impatient, ordered, "Just hurry and put her under now."

A tingling sensation started in my feet and crept up my legs. I voiced it aloud, "My legs feel funny." They asked me to count backwards from ten. I think I got as far as seven before everything went black.

Swallowed by the darkness, I floated in nothingness, in a place where time held no meaning. When I finally woke up, I desperately clung to that feeling, but it didn't last long. Although I had been told that I would wake up with a morphine drip and a button to self-administer it, there was none to be found. Perhaps that was for the best; I likely would have used it all, desperate to escape back into oblivion.

As I glanced around the bustling recovery hall, I noticed several other patients. One of them was an elderly man lying in his bed. He appeared so still and lifeless, that, for a moment, I thought he was dead, though he was probably just recovering from surgery too. The nurses bustled around, but no one seemed to notice me. I tried to lift myself up using the bed rail, but my body was too weak to respond. It wasn't until I noticed the tube between my legs that I realised a urinary catheter had been inserted, something no one had mentioned before.

Back in the ward for several days, I saw no sign of the surgeon. The consultant on the rounds couldn't even read the surgeon's notes. When I asked the nurses about my stitches, they spoke of staples, which disturbed me greatly. Three days post-surgery, I learned that I'd had open surgery, not keyhole, and no staples. The only pain relief I'd had was a paracetamol drip immediately after surgery. I didn't request any other pain relief. I told myself that if I stayed perfectly still, I wouldn't feel any pain – so I didn't move. Despite my refusal, a nurse handed me some painkillers and told me to take them so that I wouldn't "look so miserable".

The hospital food was what I expected from an underfunded, run-down community hospital. As a vegan, they gave me the same meal as everyone else, minus the meat. I grew dizzy, nauseated and weak from not eating and from sleep deprivation – thanks to the constant noise and bright lights at night. How could anyone recover in this place? The other women in the ward tried to keep their spirits up, but I stayed silent, withdrawn.

When I had another anxiety attack, despite not having eaten, I felt like I was going to vomit. When I told the nurse, she abruptly tossed a cardboard vomit pan onto my bed, without looking me in the eye. I felt like an inconvenience, a burden.

My mum tried to advocate for me, and a nurse eventually agreed to move me to a side room to recover in privacy, but no one had explained that to me. So when they wheeled me there, panic took over again. I cried out, gasping for air I couldn't seem to find. The nurses spoke about me kindly, but again, as if I wasn't there. I felt the eyes of others on me, but no one questioned why I was reacting this way. Even to this day, I blush when I think of that dramatic scene, and though I understand now why I reacted that way, I still feel mortified.

***

While in hospital, I received a phone call offering me a permanent full-time locum position with Boots, the pharmacy chain. I declined. The lack of care I'd experienced only reinforced the negative belief that I wasn't good enough. How could I work as a registered pharmacist when I felt so broken? Unemployment felt like the safer option – for everyone.

Looking back, I see that it wasn't just self-doubt that made me say no. During my time in hospital in 2011, I was re-experiencing the trauma of 2006. The student surgeon's eyes resembling those of the rapist's, and the way I was put under anesthesia without warmth or care echoed the helpless feeling of having my drink spiked by the man who raped me. Waking up paralysed, discovering the catheter between my legs, all mirrored that earlier violation.

In 2006, I struggled to speak to the A&E staff. In 2011, I cried out and was ignored. Both times, no one truly heard me. It was as if the world was too busy, too indifferent. As if the joke was on me – I was the punchline!

Chapter 22: When Worth Weighed Nothing

After my surgery, I convinced myself that I would never work in a professional capacity again. I told myself my entire four-year master's degree and post-graduate training were utterly useless, that my future would be filled with failure. And yet, I was only twenty-five. The idea of working as a pharmacist felt like a distant memory, so I ignored my mum's advice to contact a pharmacy chain that had previously offered me a job.

Months of unemployment and deepening depression brought crushing feelings of worthlessness. I spent hours ruminating over poor decisions and difficult moments from my past. I attacked every part of myself – my education, my appearance, even the fact that I'd needed surgery to remove an ovarian cyst. I fixated on these perceived flaws, which only compounded my sense of failure.

Worse still, I compared myself to peers who were advancing in their careers, travelling the world, and building strong bonds with friends and partners. I hated myself for not being able to do any of those things, for not being "normal". Scrolling through social media, the bright lives of others only deepened my isolation.

Eventually, I began applying for jobs below my skill level. After two exhausting interviews, where I fought to maintain a friendly demeanour despite the storm inside, I was offered two positions: one in a completely different industry, and one in my own. While switching industries tempted me, I was ultimately drawn to the pharmaceutical role.

At first, my confidence lifted – briefly. But nervousness and self-doubt lingered. I wasn't sure I could handle the job, let alone the daily commute. Panic attacks while driving had made me reliant on others for transportation. My new workplace was a decent distance away, and I depended on my dad for the travel to interviews and my brother for the occasional lift.

I tried to see it as a fresh start, told myself that I was open to learning. Maybe there was even a flicker of excitement about something new. But it wasn't long before my real education began – just not the kind I had expected.

Chapter 23: The Bottom of Their Shoe

I was introduced to the team as a pharmacist. I hated that. I didn't want anyone to know I was a pharmacist. Northern Ireland is a small place, and people draw conclusions quickly –whether it's based on how far apart your eyes are, how you pronounce your "H", your name, your education, your occupation, or where you live. The Troubles were over, but the cultural residue remained. There were undertones of political and religious difference that I felt but couldn't name.

Being young, autistic (though I didn't know it yet), traumatised, overqualified, and underconfident made everything harder. I could almost feel the team's suspicions – or maybe I was just a misfit. On top of that, the atmosphere at work was heavy with low morale. Colleagues smiled, but their smiles rarely reached their eyes. I quickly realised I had to work even harder to keep my mask in place. Keeping my head down wasn't enough. I told myself to focus on my work and avoid gossip. For anyone, it would have been a tough place to work. For me, it felt like a kind of living hell.

I ignored the gut feeling telling me to quit – not because I didn't hear it, but because I no longer trusted myself. I placed everyone else on a pedestal, assuming they must have it right and I must have it wrong. I convinced myself that any discomfort I felt was either my fault or imagined. So, I stayed.

But being a pharmacist seemed to attract unwanted attention. People started asking questions – lots of them. Managers from other departments began discussing plans to move me across teams. I hated it. I knew it would cause friction, and my fears were soon confirmed when subtle, negative behaviours began to appear.

One bank holiday, when most of the senior staff were off, a colleague's resentment boiled over. She lashed out at me verbally when I asked for help setting up some equipment. I reported the incident to HR, trusting they'd handle it fairly. They assured me they'd look into it and advised me to carry on working as usual.

I wasn't prepared for what followed.

I was assigned a task I hadn't been trained to complete. When I asked for help, I was refused. That final project seemed to become the reason they let me go, right at the end of my probation period. Before that decision, HR called me into a meeting that left me emotionally shattered. I was told I wasn't a good fit for the role. To make matters worse, they mentioned that the colleague who'd mistreated me was no longer with the company, as if that alone might somehow fix things.

I was devastated. I felt like nothing more than dirt beneath their shoes.

There was, however, a small glimmer of comfort: one senior manager who'd witnessed the meeting later expressed her outrage over how I'd been treated. She wanted to stay in touch and even invited me to join her for weekly Irish traditional music sessions at a local hotel. I couldn't bring myself to accept. My trust had been shattered, and I couldn't risk putting myself out there again. I still regret not replying to her.

That experience deepened my imposter syndrome and turned it into something more crippling. I felt like I had no value, that I was a burden to my family and to society. The trauma I'd experienced had led me to that job, and as the dominoes fell, I kept falling. The mistreatment, the bullying, and the way things were handled all re-triggered my trauma.

But at the time, I didn't even know I was being retraumatised. I didn't see that what was happening was part of a much larger pattern.

It was a stark reminder that no matter how far I tried to run from trauma, through a new job, a different place, or a fresh start, it followed me. The phrase "kicking someone when they're already down" doesn't even begin to describe it.

I didn't know it then, but I was dealing with PTSD. And I didn't yet understand I was autistic.

I turned inward and blamed myself. I thought I was solely responsible for everything that happened. It wasn't until more than a decade later, after another traumatic event shook my world, that I finally sought therapy.

Hope And Light

Chapter 24: Second Border Crossing, First Hope

I had convinced myself there was nothing left for me in Ireland. Though the country boasted a thriving nightlife, I wasn't part of it. By the end of 2006, I had withdrawn from the social scene almost entirely. I made rare appearances at mandatory events – birthdays, mostly – and only if I could go with family or Marek, my boyfriend at the time. Occasionally, I joined friends, but I never felt safe. My nights often ended early, punctuated by panic attacks as soon as I crawled into bed.

Unemployment weighed heavily. I couldn't drive, which left me stuck and dependent. Life in Ireland felt bleak and claustrophobic. I knew I needed change, and that change wouldn't come if I stayed. So Marek and I left for Switzerland, stopping in Italy first.

The drive from Italy into Switzerland was breathtaking. The towering Alps loomed above us – majestic, yet strangely intimidating. As I stared up at them, I was overwhelmed by a sense of insignificance. We humans are mere specks beside these ancient giants, and they, in turn, are mere specks in the vast universe. That perspective brought me moments of peace.

Landing in a place where no one knew me was exhilarating. The air was crisp, the water pure. Yes, there was a divide between locals and foreigners, but it wasn't like the divisions I'd known. Here, people from all over the world had come to make it their home.

Being close to the global pharma hub gave me hope, and I didn't have to wait long. Within months, I landed a role as a Medical Writer at a small agency. The position had originally been advertised for someone with a PhD. They chose me anyway. That offer was a huge confidence boost – I felt both thrilled and stunned.

I worked alongside PhDs, MDs, and other pharmacists in a diverse, international team. But the confidence didn't last. Imposter syndrome crept in. I told myself I was the least qualified person in the building, even though some colleagues didn't have a health sciences background at all. I placed everyone else on a pedestal, as I always had. I was afraid to ask questions. I felt out of place, unaware that this familiar feeling stretched back to 2006, when my sense of self had been fractured by the rape.

Most of my co-workers treated me kindly. But I couldn't shake the sense that some harboured unconscious bias because I lacked the PhD – a bias I likely reinforced by doubting myself. Eventually, a conflict with a male colleague tarnished my so-called fresh start. But I later learned that I wasn't the only one who struggled with him.

Regardless of those hiccups, I stayed for two years. During that time, Marek and I married, and I moved on to a new role – one that wouldn't have been possible without the experience I gained at the agency. Despite everything, something good came of it.

I realise I've skipped over my wedding. That's no oversight. There are things about that day I've yet to fully process. The ceremony took place in a small Tuscan village, surrounded by rolling hills, straight out of a film. Picture-perfect. But that fairy tale setting didn't reflect my inner world. The small guest list and distant location weren't born of romantic whimsy; they were a shield. I didn't have many people to invite, and the thought of a wedding at home filled me with dread.

Like many newlyweds, we looked forward to starting a family. We tried for nearly two years. Each month brought fresh hope, followed by crushing disappointment. Both Marek and I underwent full fertility workups. The doctors found no medical cause. Despite signs that I was ovulating, my obstetrician prescribed monthly hormone injections. They didn't work. Eventually, I gave up. She booked me in for exploratory surgery, scheduled for the week after a work trip to Rome.

Chapter 25: Sunlight Without the Shadow

I wasn't going to leave Rome, having only spent time with my work crew. So I took time in lieu, added a day or two of annual leave, and Marek eagerly flew down to meet me.

It was my third time here as a tourist, but Rome is the kind of place you never tire of. There's simply too much to see. The cobbled streets branch into more cobbled streets, forming a web of alleys filled with surprises – architectural gems and ancient ruins, beauty around every corner. The city is a feast for the senses, and we savoured it all.

It was spring – perfect for outdoor pleasures. We sat at the edge of a piazza with an aperitivo, delighting in focaccia, olives, crisps, and tickling ourselves giddy with a Prosecco or spritz. This was the life. And it felt even better knowing we were in Rome with the strength of our Swiss franc – we could spoil ourselves without worry.

I remember telling Marek one evening, as I swirled my Chianti in its wide glass at the end of our meal, that perhaps it wasn't so bad, after all, having no children. Maybe this was meant to be. I could get used to this easy-going lifestyle.

That evening ended early. I felt unusually tired, but after days of meetings, presentations, team-building, and now sightseeing, it was no surprise. We went to bed early, ready for the Vatican the next day.

Chapter 26: Sanctified and Silenced

We visited the Vatican as planned. At one point, we found ourselves sitting outside a row of confessional booths. We were simply tired and needed a rest, but we soon realised confessions were taking place. I joked that we should go in. Marek didn't realise I was joking.

"It would be a truly memorable experience if we did," he said.

I was unconvinced. I hadn't been to confession in years – not since childhood. But Marek kept nudging me. "If you go, I'll go."

I had no intention of going in. I was quite happy to wait for him. When he emerged, proud of himself, he kept encouraging me. I remember thinking, *If I don't do this, I'll never hear the end of it.*

Reluctantly, I stepped into the booth.

When the priest asked what I wanted to confess, I froze. This was a stranger, not a native English speaker, and I couldn't even see his face. But somehow, I stumbled into words, speaking of my struggles to conceive, the heartache of watching others build families.

I hadn't expected to go so deep. Even as I spoke, I remember thinking, *Why couldn't I have just said I took the Lord's name in vain and left it at that?*

A silence followed. Then the priest suggested that perhaps I didn't deserve children. That God had decided I was unworthy, and I should consider adopting a spiritual child instead.

His words hit me like a slap. I left the booth in tears, my chest burning with rage. But I swallowed it down. All around me, tourists and worshippers admired golden ceilings and priceless art. I wanted to scream. I even considered writing a letter to the Pope.

New Beginnings

Chapter 27: A Lease of New Life

The flight from Rome to Zurich was short, but the evening felt long. It seemed to take forever to get back to Luzern. When we finally got home, we collapsed into bed and drifted off almost instantly.

But in the early hours, I woke, restless and uneasy. Then it came to me – the spotting I'd noticed a couple of days earlier, the assumption that it signalled yet another disappointing month. But my period hadn't arrived.

At 5 a.m., I took a pregnancy test. Positive.

I shook Marek awake, breathless with excitement. He insisted I take another. Positive again.

We were having a baby.

No spiritual child needed.

No surgery needed.

We had a new lease on life, and from that moment, I have never slept quite the same.

Chapter 28: The Weight Beneath the Cradle

The next chapter of our lives began. I stayed with my job until the contract ended, and nine months and nine days later, our son was born. The company offered me a full-time position, but they wanted me back when he was just fourteen weeks old. I couldn't do it. Leaving a newborn in daycare felt unimaginable. I was still breastfeeding constantly. Exhausted. Raw. Completely devoted. It was a decision made from love, not fear – and I have never doubted it.

But I quickly became a lonely new mum in a foreign country, unable to speak the local language, with no family nearby. The weight of motherhood hit hard. I never got over the shock. While Marek was at work, I stayed home, cocooned with my son, anxious and overwhelmed.

I blamed myself for not being like the other mums, who seemed to glide effortlessly through early motherhood. Even now, seven years on, I still struggle.

Marek and our midwife noticed my anxiety, but no one grasped how severe it was. I was seriously unwell, and the lack of support only deepened my isolation. My experience of motherhood was clouded by fear, self-doubt, and sadness. It strained my relationship with Marek and complicated my ability to bond with my son. I believe it affected him too. Trauma is contagious – it moves between bodies like a virus.

When trauma strikes, it changes everything. There is no reset button for the brain. I didn't know I had PTSD, so I didn't understand the triggers that shaped my everyday life. Looking back, I believe that if the rape in 2006 had never happened, I might have handled pregnancy, birth, and early motherhood very differently.

I might have conceived sooner. Our fertility tests found no physical issues. The emotional toll was the likely culprit.

The mind and body are deeply connected. No matter how hard I tried to build a life, it always felt as if I was swimming against a current too strong to fight.

Chapter 29: Settling Down

It took time for Marek and me to agree on moving back to Ireland. It was one of the hardest decisions we ever faced. We had grown used to the Swiss lifestyle: fresh Alpine air, crystal-clear lake swims in summer, crisp hikes in spring and autumn, and our first ski lessons in winter. The healthcare system was in a different league from what we knew in Italy or Ireland. The strong economy and financial comfort still felt new to us, even after seven years.

Despite all that, we lived modestly, renting a small two-bedroom apartment that allowed us to save. But money wasn't everything. What we lacked, and deeply missed, was family. We didn't want to raise our son surrounded by values that didn't fully align with our own. We wanted him close to loved ones, especially my mum.

We debated: stay in Switzerland, or return to Ireland? Once we reflected on our values, the answer became clear. The sooner we moved home, the better.

Just as we began taking steps, the pandemic hit. Everything became more complicated. We experienced lockdown in three countries: Switzerland, Italy, and Ireland. It was eye-opening. The contrasts in how governments, cultures, and communities responded were stark. Things we had never noticed before became glaringly obvious.

House-hunting was a challenge. Being abroad limited our options, and Northern Irish mortgage lenders weren't eager to help. Still, we found a three-bedroom semi-detached house just a six-minute walk from my parents' home. They viewed it for us, sending photos and videos. Trusting our instincts – and with the help of our Swiss nest egg – we made one of our bravest decisions: we bought it sight unseen.

We left Switzerland as quietly as we had once left Ireland. In the summer of 2020, we returned to Newry, County Down. Everything began to fall into place. Family nearby. Familiar faces. Our son would grow up knowing his maternal grandparents. For the first time in a long time, I could exhale. The tension lifted. Life finally felt normal.

With our son preparing to start nursery, I saw a chance to return to the career path I'd begun before pregnancy. I applied for jobs, braced myself for rejection, and stayed open to whatever came next. We were finally settling down.

Chapter 30: When Love Kept Me Alive

"Love is not a victory march, it's a cold and it's a broken hallelujah."

— LEONARD COHEN

By autumn 2020, we had moved into our new home. For the first time in years, I felt a sense of calm – a new normal. It wasn't adventurous, but it was quietly blissful. Mum would take my son for a few hours now and then, giving Marek and me rare moments together. I started doing ordinary things with Mum again, the sort of everyday pleasures daughters often take for granted – lunches out, walks along Greenan Road. Colour was returning to my life.

And then, just as we settled into this gentle rhythm, everything changed. Mum fell ill. What followed devastated us. The details are too raw to share here – I've spoken of them while volunteering for Pancreatic Cancer UK's Optimal Care Pathway and in interviews on regional and national TV news. What I didn't realise then was that each time I spoke publicly, I was reclaiming a voice I had lost at nineteen, maybe even earlier. Speaking out about my mum was liberating, but it was shattering.

Her cancer journey was brutal. The trauma affected us all deeply. In June 2021, our beautiful mum passed away in Daisy Hill Hospital, Newry. My family and I cared for her right to the end, watching her take her final breaths. I will never get over the agony of losing her, nor the journey that preceded it. I'm not sure I've even begun to grieve. There's too much unprocessed pain, too much complex trauma.

This wasn't the life I envisioned when we came home. People still offer condolences, kindly reminding me how lucky I was to be home in time to care for her. Maybe it was a blessing. But behind my polite smile, I often feel the opposite: profoundly unlucky.

Mum was meant to care for my son so I could return to work. That same week her cancer was discovered, I was offered an excellent job. I turned it down without hesitation. I've never regretted that choice, but I do resent the cruel twist of fate that made it necessary.

I know many others suffer too, and my heart breaks for them, but that doesn't lessen our pain. Each family bears its own unbearable grief.

The day after Mum's burial, I woke with searing, stabbing pain from head to toe, as if every cell in my body was screaming. I'd never felt anything like it. I thought it was COVID, but there was no fever, no cough. I spent the day in bed except for thirty minutes when I forced myself up to take my son to his nursery graduation. What should have been a joyful milestone, one Mum would have shared with us, was a blur of physical agony and emotional numbness.

It confirmed something I'd long suspected: trauma doesn't just haunt the mind. It embeds itself in the body.

That thought stayed with me.

A few months later, in Italy, I lay on a bed, staring up at the thick wooden beams. I imagined myself hanging from one. And then, in a moment of piercing clarity, I pictured my four-year-old son finding me. That image stopped me cold. I knew, then and there, that something had to change. My mother's death had shattered what remained of me. I needed help, and I finally accepted it.

I opened my laptop and sent the email:

6 August 2021

Hello,

I would like to enquire regarding appointments for psychotherapy with David. What is his availability, and how much do sessions cost?

Kind regards,

Journey To Justice

Awakening and Research

Chapter 31: Locking Doors

I often carry the heavy burden of feeling responsible for not being strong enough to cope with situations others believe I *should* be able to handle. Even though I know the total loss of control I experienced when my drink was spiked and I was violated wasn't my fault, that feeling still lingers. My automatic defences decided how I would respond to the attack; I had no power to change the outcome. This man set out to hurt me, and there was nothing I could do to stop him.

It wouldn't have happened if I hadn't been in the wrong place at the wrong time. Actually, I should rephrase that, because that still sounds like I'm blaming myself. *It wouldn't have happened if he hadn't been there.* This was my family home, and I *was* in the right place at the right time. That's what makes the injury feel even more profound. He was a stranger who had either been innocently invited by someone in our circle or who had purposefully entered the premises himself.

It took me a long time to comprehend that none of this was in my control. I've come to understand that it wasn't my fault, but knowing that doesn't lessen the impact of the trauma. That night, Newry stopped feeling like a safe place. From then on, I began to close off, locking doors – both literally and metaphorically.

Chapter 32: The Panic They Called "Personality"

In my daily life, I still get triggered, even when my rational mind insists there's no danger. That's the cruelty of PTSD: once triggered, the brain bypasses logic and defaults to survival mode, just as it did during the original trauma. When that switch flips, I'm no longer in the present. I'm back there – in the aftermath of the assault, or worse, reliving the terror as if it's happening all over again.

In a world steeped in toxic positivity, managing these episodes has been incredibly difficult. Until I understood what they were, I believed they were just part of me – a personal failing. I thought I wasn't coping as well as everyone else. Slogans like "man up", "bounce back", and "it's all about resilience" cut deep. How do you "pull yourself together" when your body is reacting with the force of an injury, involuntary and overwhelming, like a seizure? Until therapy, I didn't even know I was being triggered.

The response to a trigger goes far beyond what most people think of as anxiety. It's like calmly walking along a canal and being shoved from behind into deep, freezing water – sudden, jarring, terrifying. Fear skyrockets from zero to one hundred in an instant. I can go from feeling relatively content to full-blown panic in a heartbeat. The shaking, the intense heat and cold, the sweating, the churning stomach, the frantic breathing – at its height, it feels like it will never end. Sometimes the only "relief", and I use that word cautiously, comes after vomiting, often repeatedly.

This isn't fear over something that *might* happen. It's a reaction to something that *has already happened*. Something brutal. Something that carved itself into my body and my life. And yet it's deeply isolating, because most people cannot grasp it. Instead,

I'm labelled: anxious, dramatic, panicky over nothing. These labels erase the truth – that what you're seeing is a visceral, automatic response born of trauma.

When someone tells me to "snap out of it" or gently says "you're okay", it compounds the harm. Because in those moments, *I'm not okay.*

The aftermath of these episodes is challenging in a different way. I'm left completely drained. Basic self-care becomes hard. Recovery can take days, sometimes weeks. When trauma goes unacknowledged and triggers are unrecognised, it feels like being silenced all over again.

Everything began to change when I started analytical therapy. The trauma was finally acknowledged. I began to understand what was happening in my body and mind. I'm deeply grateful to my Nexus counsellor, who taught me practical techniques to manage episodes. And in analytical therapy with David, I worked on identifying my triggers. Sometimes, simply acknowledging a trigger as it arises is enough to stop it from spiralling. And when fear shows its grim face again, I try to practise what Nexus taught me. Often, it's enough to prevent the panic from escalating. When an episode does take hold, despite all my efforts, I remind myself of everything I've learned from both David and Nexus. I can name it now. I know what it is. And I know it *will* pass.

Therapy has helped reduce the number of episodes – in 2022 and 2023, they dropped significantly. But since reporting the rape, the attacks have crept back in. As long as the case remains open and unresolved, it feels like my healing is suspended. He may no longer be physically present, but his refusal to admit what he did still seeps into my life, prolonging the pain, not just for me, but for my family too.

That's why it enrages me when courts reduce sentences for perpetrators who only confess when they're cornered. What about the years we lose while they deny, delay, and drag us through the so-called justice system? The trauma of the assault is already unbearable. The system should never deepen that pain. And yet, it does.

Chapter 33: Holy Before I Was Whole

Therapy took me on a journey – one that explored thought processes and emotional landscapes I had never consciously examined before. It was often turbulent and challenging, not least because of the emotional bricks I'd laid over the years to wall off certain experiences. But as I dismantled those bricks, piece by piece, I began uncovering thoughts and feelings that had long been buried or dismissed. There was no clear order to it. Most days, I found myself jumping between emotions: shame, denial, sadness, worthlessness, acceptance, and, eventually, forgiveness.

As I wrestled with these feelings and came to terms with the fact that I had been raped, my focus shifted towards the rapist himself. Maybe this was a defence mechanism – a way to avoid the raw pain of what his violence had done to me.

Despite navigating this inner storm, I still had to keep moving through the rhythms of everyday life. I had a child, a husband, responsibilities. Life didn't stop. But becoming a mother offered me a new lens on my past. Watching my son grow, so full of intelligence, beauty, and potential, I clung to a powerful belief: no one is born evil.

And so the question began to haunt me: *What had happened to him?* What turned him into someone capable of rape? Why did he do this to me?

For someone with an autistic mind, unanswered questions can feel unbearable. I sought answers, hoping to find peace through understanding. Motherhood had taught me a fundamental truth: every human being needs love. Through my reading, particularly the work of Dr Gabor Maté, I saw how trauma, especially the absence of love and connection, can shape a person's path.

I asked myself: If I were to withhold love from my son, what might become of him? Could a lack of love drive someone to harm others? Was the man who raped me unloved too? Had his rage grown in that absence?

When I turned my gaze inward, I often felt like "damaged goods" – worthless because of what had been done to me. But over time, I saw the truth: *he* was the damaged one. His violence wasn't just an act; it was a transmission of his own brokenness, passed onto me. I carried that pain as if it were mine.

In that realisation, I came to see him, however painfully, as someone who may once have been a hurting, unloved child. That understanding doesn't excuse what he did. Nothing can. Adults know right from wrong. They know the law. Trauma never justifies inflicting trauma on others.

Yet still, in quiet moments, I sometimes saw him not only as a rapist but as a human being who had once been innocent. That brought a complicated mix of sorrow and compassion. And sometimes, compassion became something even more startling: love. It was through these moments of compassion that forgiveness became imaginable.

For me, forgiveness is not possible without compassion. And compassion, at its most distilled, is a form of love.

As I moved toward forgiveness – through grief, confusion, empathy, and fear – I came to believe that true healing would only come by facing him. Meeting him. Looking him in the eye. Not to excuse or forget, but to reclaim my story. Forgiveness gave me the strength to even consider that possibility.

But as I reflect on this journey, I now recognise that one essential emotion remained unacknowledged: **anger**.

Anger – righteous, protective, powerful – had not yet fully claimed its place.

Where was it?

Chapter 34: Texting the Devil

As I continued working through the mental and emotional aspects of my treatment for rape trauma, an idea began to form – both absurd and, somehow, deeply necessary: *What would it be like to meet the man who had caused all this pain?*

So, I did what I've always done in moments of uncertainty: I researched. I needed to know if it was okay to want to meet my rapist. Looking back, I think my autism played a significant role in this process, though at the time, I hadn't yet been diagnosed.

Like many autistic individuals, I had spent most of my life masking, learning "social rules" by mimicking others. I observed people in my life, copied what I saw on TV or read in books, and tried to adapt. But I'm only now realising that sometimes I applied these rules incorrectly, in ways that didn't align with neurotypical expectations. It's like trying to compare an Apple device with an Android – my wiring is simply different. For much of my life, I was measured against a neurotypical standard, and that caused me significant distress. This distress was often misunderstood. I had spent years stumbling and fumbling through life in ways my neurotypical counterparts never had to experience.

So when I found myself unsure about whether meeting my rapist was the right thing to do, I researched it. I needed to understand if this was something others had done, if it was a legitimate path to healing, and – perhaps most importantly – if it was okay for me to even consider it. I didn't feel comfortable speaking about this idea aloud, fearing judgment, misunderstanding, and perhaps even disbelief.

It was during this research that I came across a TED Talk by an Icelandic woman, Thordis Elva. She had been 16 years old when she was raped by an Australian exchange student in her home-town. In her talk, Thordis shared her powerful story, where she spoke about how she ultimately forgave her rapist. What struck me most was that she chose to reach out to him, travelling across the globe to meet him in Cape Town. During their meeting, they spoke openly, reconciled, and remained in contact afterwards. Her rapist expressed genuine remorse, and through this encounter, Thordis found a sense of healing.[10]

I was deeply moved by her story, especially the idea of confronting the person who had caused so much trauma and finding healing in the process. I later learned that this type of meeting is called "restorative justice". While I hadn't known the term before, I understood that restorative justice is typically carried out within a structured environment, often with professional oversight and support. To this day, I still don't know if such a service is offered in Northern Ireland.

However, I felt driven by the same motivations that guide victims who seek restorative justice. In my case, I was attempting to initiate this process on my own. Inspired by Thordis Elva's example, I believed that I, too, could meet my rapist and perhaps find some kind of healing in the process. So I decided to track him down.

I took a leap, posting anonymously in a Facebook group for lost family and friends, asking if anyone knew him and could put us in contact. Although he didn't have a social media profile that I was aware of, there were people who knew him online, and it didn't take long before someone responded. This person acted as a go-between, facilitating contact between us.

I had found him.

Now that I had located him, the next question was: What was I supposed to do now?

---

10 Elva, T. (2023, March 27). Thordis Elva discusses why she waived her right to anonymity as a rape survivor [Video]. YouTube. https://www.youtube.com/watch?v=gyPoqFcvt9w

Revisiting the Past

Chapter 35: Swept Away by the Rip Tide

Seventeen years had passed since that night—the night that man became part of my story without my consent. I hadn't seen him since. Then, in 2022, I reached out. He seemed a bit spooked by the unexpected contact, but he was eager to meet up as soon as possible. Just days later, we met in a hotel in the Newry and Mourne area.

I had wanted to meet in the lobby – it felt safer: open, with chairs placed at a distance and the reception desk in my line of sight. But he texted to say he was in the bar. When I read the message, my heart pounded, and I literally jumped out of my seat. Fear washed over me, and my logical brain shut down. I wanted this over with. Without taking a moment, I walked straight towards the bar. From the moment I saw him, I froze again.

Physically, he was a large man – much larger than I – but not as imposing as he had seemed in 2006. Back then, the fear had shrunk me so much that everyone around me, especially him, seemed towering. But I wasn't that small person anymore. I had grown. Through counselling, I was becoming the size I am, slowly rebuilding my self-worth. I noticed that he had aged, gained some weight, but his eyes – those same eyes – remained unchanged.

With a forced smile that barely concealed his discomfort, he stretched his arms out to hug me, as if we were old friends. I felt vulnerable, but my mind could not process what was happening fast enough. My defences kicked in, and I defaulted to "friend" mode, awkwardly making a half attempt at a light, distant hug – just to get through that part and move on to the real reason for meeting. It took months more of therapy to understand why I responded that way, why I instinctively fawned and friended.

He led the way into the bar, and my legs followed, carrying me along. Though the location wasn't my choice, I felt somewhat safer knowing there were people around, even if only a few. In hindsight, though, I realise he had the upper hand – he had steered us to the bar when I had wanted to stay in the lounge. From there, I became hyper-aware of myself. I chose a seat next to another woman, just to feel some proximity to safety.

As I sat down, I tried to cut straight to the point. "I'm sure you're wondering what this is all about, so I want to get straight to it."

He quickly interrupted, asking – word for word – "Is this about consent?"

I was stunned. Just minutes into seeing him again, and he was already bringing up consent. *Consent.* My mind reeled. Why would he ask that unless he knew he was guilty? Why would he drive for over an hour, after all these years, to meet me, and then bring up consent if he had nothing to hide?

Once I confirmed that, yes, I wanted to talk about consent, the conversation quickly spiralled. He hijacked it, listing one reason after another why I wouldn't be believed. The level of detail in his explanations – the different angles he presented – all felt like well-researched arguments. I hadn't prepared for this. I could not process it. The barrage of his words overwhelmed me.

As he continued listing reasons, his questions turned personal, probing into my medical records. I felt nausea rise in my throat. I tried to respond, but when I did, he couldn't even look at me. His gaze darted all around the room, distracted, uneasy. His nervousness was so obvious – yet it felt disproportionate to the crushing anxiety I felt inside. My body trembled, as if my very insides were quaking. My hands and feet felt like ice blocks. A wave of worthlessness coursed through me.

Without giving me the chance to challenge him, he abruptly suggested we go to the nearest police station to "sort things out there". Even though I didn't see it at the time, he was using every ounce of his manipulation and intimidation skills to make me question my own perceptions of reality.

Amid his anxious glances over his shoulder, he insisted we move to the other side of the bar. He believed the woman sitting near us was eavesdropping. I agreed to move. At that moment, I could only handle one fight – the fight to confront him about how he had raped me, twice. But physically, I felt sick, drained, and I needed to conserve what little strength I had left.

I had no idea he was actively gaslighting me in the same way he had in 2006, when he pursued me for weeks after the assault. If I had known then what I know now, I would have walked away. But fear overtook my logical mind, and I defaulted to what I knew: appease him. Keep him calm. Keep him on my side, because that was the only way I knew to protect myself.

I reassured him, telling him I would never report what happened and that I had no interest in going to the police. At that moment, I genuinely believed it was the best course of action. Nothing would come of it anyway – or so I thought.

As the meeting wore on, I found myself drifting further from my body. The overwhelming flood of fear pulled me into dissociation. He absorbed my trauma response – my fawning and my appeasing behaviour – and used it to his advantage. He denied everything I said. He didn't listen to how his actions had affected me. Instead, he pontificated, avoiding eye contact, clearing his throat repeatedly, his body language shifty and evasive, telling me how he would never have done something like that.

Then he turned the conversation again. He told me how difficult his life had been, launching into a detailed story about sinister experiences from his past. He had me – but something deep inside me didn't trust any of it. He even cried, and I was caught in a fog of confusion, torn between what might be real and what might not. They felt like crocodile tears. And somehow, despite knowing better, I found myself feeling sorry for him. I felt sorry for the man who had raped me. I felt sorry for him because he'd made such an effort to travel down to meet me. For a moment, it was as if *I* had done something wrong. His feelings – full of lies and manipulation – overshadowed my own. While I wasn't conscious of it at the time, I felt violated once more.

Being in his presence again made me question my own perception of reality. I questioned my sanity. There was a deep conflict between what I felt and what I thought, between what I knew and what I was being made to believe. I left that meeting wanting to die.

Even though, from the moment I saw him, my denial about what had happened to me was finally shattered, I still could not shake the feeling that I was somehow to blame. My empathy for him, feeling sorry for him, drowned out any anger that was trying to surface. Seeing him in the flesh brought it all rushing back. He raped me. There was no denying it now. But somehow, all the work I had done in therapy up until that point felt undone by being in his presence.

That meeting was a wake-up call: I should never doubt myself again. And yet, in that moment, I felt completely destroyed by the encounter. When I returned home that Saturday afternoon, I wanted nothing more than to be locked away – far from the world, far from the pain.

Looking back, I now realise I had fallen prey to a textbook narcissistic gaslighter. He was a master manipulator. I sensed he knew he was guilty. I knew he was guilty. And I felt that he knew I knew.

He raped me – and he carried himself with a sort of confidence, as if he believed there was nothing I could do about it. I had pledged to him, and to myself, that I would not report him. But when I got home, I was left with an overwhelming sense of regret. I stumbled upstairs, put on my pyjamas, and curled up on the couch, pulling a heavy throw around me. Suicidal thoughts crept in, and I couldn't help but wonder: *What kind of person chooses to meet with their rapist?*

Marek spent the day keeping my son entertained, and the only person I wanted to speak with was David. But Wednesday's session felt like an eternity away.

Chapter 36: Only Poison Matched the Pain

After our meeting at the hotel, my healing process continued – but not in a straight line. I got worse before I got better. In those early stages, my mental health deteriorated rapidly. Thirteen days later, on a midweek evening, I found myself completely overwhelmed by an unbearable wave of anxiety. Desperate for relief, I reached for something deeply personal and symbolic: my late mother's THC oil, a potent herbal extract she had used during her cancer journey.

Using it was entirely out of character for me. As an autistic pharmacist, I am meticulous about what I put into my body, and turning to an illegal, psychoactive substance went against everything I stood for, although I had already been challenged in this area when my mother was dying of cancer, and its use was suggested. However, that night, I simply couldn't cope; I could find no relief from the torturous amount of anxiety I felt.

What followed was an unintentional drug trip – my first, and hopefully my last. Instead of calming me, the THC did the exact opposite. The panic hit like a freight train. My heart raced uncontrollably, my chest burned as if it were on fire, and my blood pressure soared. I spiralled into an intense, prolonged panic attack, and the paramedics wouldn't leave me until my blood pressure and heart rate fell. They asked what had triggered the anxiety and while I admitted that I had consumed THC, I could not bring myself to tell them why I had taken it – that it was my attempt to self-medicate and manage the severe anxiety that only escalated following a recent meeting with the man who raped me. Even in my drugged state, a paralysing fear gripped me. I was terrified they would report it to the police. So, I told them I was grieving the loss of my mother. And while that was true, it wasn't the full story. Her death had deeply affected me, but it was the trauma I was still processing that had brought me to this point.

The following day I had called my GPs and told them about the episode and the use of THC and had asked for help to manage my anxiety, a level of which had clearly spiralled out of control. I also addressed the issue with David. I never again tried to self-medicate illegally; that night showed me that path only led to more harm.

In the weeks and months that followed, that episode forced me to reflect on its true cause. I began to replay the meeting, examining both the spoken words and the non-verbal communication that had passed between us. It took time, but eventually I came to terms with something that had unsettled me from the start: despite my compassionate and open-hearted approach, he had shown no remorse.

At moments during that meeting, I had felt forgiveness. But that forgiveness was gradually interrupted – and at times overtaken – by anger. As I processed what had happened, I realised something deeply disturbing: this man seemed experienced in what he did, from the rape itself to his behaviour following the rape. And that led me to a disturbing question: *How many others might there be?*

It was this question that, weeks later, left me wondering: *Should I report the crime?*

Chapter 37: Googling Justice

While I had begun to process the meeting with the rapist, it took a long time for me to fully comprehend the degree of manipulation and gaslighting I had been subjected to. Once I truly understood this, anger festered further. How could I have been so foolish as to let him control me like that?

I didn't want to make any more mistakes, but that's difficult when you're an undiagnosed autistic person and everything feels like a challenge. What is considered "neurotypical" or "normal" doesn't feel normal or natural to someone like me. So, I turned to research, because I had no idea how to report a non-recent crime or what to expect. The whole process of reporting a crime was foreign to me. Like many neurodivergent individuals facing unfamiliar situations, I thought research would be my best bet.

During my search, I came across Sexual Offences Legal Advisers (SOLAs). At first, I thought this was fantastic – legal representation for rape victims. I couldn't pass up the opportunity, so I called them. I imagined I'd speak with someone right away, but instead, I was placed on a waiting list. "Great, more waiting," I thought. "I'll probably change my mind by the time they call me."

When they eventually did call back, I learned that SOLAs weren't the legal support I had hoped for. They weren't there to offer the kind of in-depth advocacy a victim deserves. Instead, SOLAs are government-funded solicitors who provide virtual support. They explained that their role was to help with the administrative side of the criminal justice process, but they could not discuss the specifics of my case. They walked me through how to report the crime and what the criminal justice process would look like. They also mentioned the grim statistics of the incredibly low conviction rates.

I hung up the phone feeling utterly deflated. I had to ask myself: *Was it worth putting myself through this process if the chances of a conviction were so slim?* And if I did decide to report the crime, could I go through it without the same legal protections and support the defence would have? At this point in my decision-making process, I really felt like there was no incentive to report the crime. Yet, this man was still out there, free to do as he pleased in our society, potentially victimising others. Nothing about the situation felt right. I was left feeling insecure and uncertain, with so many unanswered questions.

Systematic Struggles

Chapter 38: He Has Lawyers, Victims Have Truth

The SOLA informed me of a shocking reality: in rape cases in the UK, it's the Crown vs the defendant, not the victim vs the defendant. The complainant is referred to as a witness, not a victim. As a witness, I realised I would be treated like anyone else – a bystander to the crime, rather than the person who suffered it. If the Public Prosecution Service (PPS) in Northern Ireland took my case to court, the defence would challenge my credibility, because that's what they do with all witnesses.

The thought of being publicly scrutinised, having my entire story questioned in front of a jury, made my insides twist. As an autistic person, I had spent a lifetime battling self-doubt, feeling judged, and struggling with misunderstandings. The idea of enduring this process, having my credibility tested in a courtroom, made me feel vulnerable. On top of that, I had to accept that my case wasn't truly mine. The Crown would be the one prosecuting, not me. Being a "witness" instead of a victim felt like another layer of separation, a barrier to reporting the crime. It left me yearning for a logical explanation – some reason that would make sense of the absurdity of it all.

Even more discouraging was learning that legal representation is only a privilege granted to the defendant. If I were a victim of any other crime – say, a car crash caused by a drunk driver – I'd be entitled to legal help. But not in cases of rape. The double standard in the criminal justice system was glaring. The alleged rapist would have at least a solicitor, or at most a team of lawyers at his disposal, offering guidance on everything: what to say, what not to say, how to frame his responses. He would be prepped, coached, and advised. His voice – but his lawyer's words – would be the ones the jury would hear. Meanwhile, my evidence, my raw, unfiltered words, would be all I had. No legal representative to guide or protect me.

It was maddening. I couldn't help but wonder: What happened to the oath to "tell the whole truth and nothing but the truth"? In this system, it was only the victim who was expected to uphold that oath. Meanwhile, the defendant's coached response was deemed acceptable – authentic, even. If I had been coached, I'd be accused of untruthful testimony. It seemed as though justice had been twisted into something unrecognisable. Perhaps, I thought, rape was effectively decriminalised here – if not in the letter of the law, then in the practice of it.

As I absorbed all of this, a clear, silent message seemed to echo through the legal system: *Do not report. It's not worth it.* It was powerful – disheartening. But I refused to accept it. My research continued, driven by the need to find a reason to report this crime, to justify the effort. I needed something, anything, that could offer hope. I searched for a rationale, something that would explain this absurd legal system. *Maybe there are many false reports,* I thought. *Maybe that's the reason they make it so hard to obtain justice. Perhaps that was the missing piece.*

Chapter 39: Imagined Injustice Screams Louder Than the Real One

I was like a dog with a bone. My autistic special interest turned into obsessively researching UK rape crime statistics. I discovered that less than 2 per cent of reported rapes result in a conviction.[11] *What happens to the other 98 per cent?* Could they all be false allegations? If I could understand this, maybe I could forgive the system and work with it. I needed to understand why the system seemed to protect the perpetrator and leave the victim unprotected – a system that, over time, I had become all too familiar with but hadn't fully recognised before. Solving this puzzle became an urgent need for me, perhaps tied to unresolved childhood trauma I wasn't yet aware of as I pored over the statistics.

The only theory I could come up with to excuse the system was the possibility of a significant number of false allegations. That might explain the "mass public anxiety" – the fear that an innocent man could be jailed for something he didn't do. It would explain why the system seemed so intent on protecting the accused. But when I dug into the Home Office statistics, my theory was shattered. The public anxiety was unfounded.

My emotions soared as I read on. I felt a deep, simmering anger. The disproportionate concern over the possibility of wrongly convicting an innocent man, versus the real need to obtain justice for rape victims, was not just unjustifiable – it was actively harming victims like me. I imagined that this fear had become entrenched in the jury system, with jurors reflecting the anxieties of the wider society. The numbers on false allegations should have been enough to put those fears to rest. Why hadn't they?

---

11 Saunders Law. "Virtually All Rape Victims Are Denied Justice – Here Is the Roadmap to Failure." Saunders & Co., https://www.saunders.co.uk/news/virtually-all-rape-victims-are-denied-justice-here-is-the-roadmap-to-failure

The numbers were clear. While figures on false allegations vary slightly, they remain consistently low.[12] According to Home Office research, only 4 per cent of sexualised violence and rape reports in the UK are found or suspected to be false. In Europe and the U.S., the figures are even lower, around 2 per cent and 6 per cent, respectively. What's even more troubling is that these statistics are often inflated. Police sometimes label cases as "no crime" or "unfounded" when they cannot gather sufficient corroborating evidence. But this doesn't mean the reports were false; it simply means there wasn't enough evidence to proceed. These two things – false reports and insufficient evidence – are often grouped together, misleadingly inflating the false allegations figure.

My mind raced, overwhelmed by the contradiction. The statistics were clear: victims tell the truth. Yet, the criminal justice system systematically protects the defendant and leaves victims out in the cold. I already felt left out in the cold – and I hadn't even reported the crime!

It made me question why society wasn't enraged by the abysmal rape conviction rates. Rapists are released without conviction, free to offend again. They could be sitting among us – friends, neighbours, colleagues, even family. At times, it feels as though rape is treated differently than other serious crimes: under-prosecuted and under-supported. Worse still, I later learned that unless charged, a rapist's anonymity can be protected for up to 25 years after their death.[13]

As victims, we are left to face this already lonely ordeal alone. This legal system deters people from reporting at all. Who would want to endure the pain of reporting a crime when there's only a 2 per

---

12 The Open University. "False Accusations of Sexual Violence: Research Summary." Open University Research, https://research.open.ac.uk/news/false-accusations-sexual-violence

13 BBC News. (2023, September 27). Northern Ireland: Pre-charge bail limit extended to 9 months. https://www.bbc.co.uk/news/uk-northern-ireland-66942145

cent chance of a conviction? I thought about walking away and moving on with my life. And for a while, that's exactly what I did.

Voice and Truth

Chapter 40: The Truth Wouldn't Let Me Sleep

Moving on with my life and forgetting the whole ordeal was harder than I expected. Thoughts crept in at all hours, uninvited. Had I made the right choice? Could I truly move on? I was torn, the decision gnawing at my insides, my mind echoing the voices of others: *It's not worth reporting, Anna. Just move on with your life.*

They were right in some ways. My case would never go anywhere. But the nagging tension in my chest – a quiet, persistent pull – told me I couldn't ignore this feeling. The body never lies. When words fail us, when our voices are silenced, our bodies speak the truth.

I'd spent most of my adult life battling anxiety and panic attacks – my body's way of communicating what I couldn't say. For years, I'd ignored my instincts, pushing them aside in favour of what others told me to do, measuring myself against a neurotypical standard. But now, it was harder to silence that inner voice. David had helped me learn to listen to my needs, to trust the voice within. Still, I wasn't satisfied with the decision to remain silent, to not report the crime.

The odds were against me, but could I live with myself knowing a rapist was still out there? Could I forgive myself for not trying to make the streets a little safer? What if, years from now, I changed my mind and it was too late – he was dead, or dying? What if I reported him and he came after me? Was my family safe? I believed he had spiked my drink; he had already hurt me – what else was he capable of?

What if there were others? Could I move on in good conscience, knowing he might hurt someone else? Would I be the first to report him, or had others already tried? Could my report be the one that led to his arrest, or would it just sit in a file?

My mind was a storm of questions. I needed professional support, but lawyers don't consult with victims, unless it's the morning of or a day before the case is heard in court. SOLAs helped, but they couldn't advise on the specific challenges of my case. So where could I turn for help? With so many unanswered questions, there was no peace. I lay awake through long, sleepless nights, dragging myself through the exhausting days. I tried to calm myself, tried to rest, but my mind wouldn't let me.

Chapter 41: What I Already Knew

One typical midweek evening, after tucking in my son, I settled onto the sofa in my pyjamas, my feet on Marek's lap, a soft blanket over us both. This was our usual routine – a quiet, comforting break to de-stress after a long day. As parents to a child with additional needs, we rarely spoke much in the evenings; we were too tired.

But that night felt different. We were about to start a Netflix series, but I couldn't focus. My mind raced with questions and *what ifs*.

I started asking Marek some of the things I'd asked many times before. I could tell he was growing weary of my torment. He sighed and said gently, "Anna, you're tormenting yourself. The only way to put an end to this agony is to report it."

In that moment, I knew he was right. His reassurance shifted something within me. I leaned closer to the decision. I was going to report the crime. But when? It's not every day you call 101 to report rape. I didn't want to rush the most important decision of my life. I'd already waited this long, so taking another week or two felt like a way to do it on my terms.

Chapter 42: Crumbs, Clarity, and Courage

As a wife, mother, sister, daughter, and niece, I worried about the burden I'd bring onto my family. Even with Marek's full support, we were already grieving and struggling – just the two of us, parenting an autistic child, still reeling from my mum's death. Life was hard enough.

If I were to report this, we couldn't do it alone. But therapy had taught me there's strength in asking for help, and I knew I had to lean into that.

Through online research and anonymous posts on a local Facebook group, I found some support. I learned, following a trail of crumbs, that much of today's support for rape victims only became available after the rugby rape trials in Ireland. Those trials exposed how the justice system often favoured perpetrators, leaving victims re-traumatised. The public outrage sparked a review of laws and procedures for serious sexual offences in Northern Ireland. But like all media storms, attention faded.[14,15]

Thankfully, charities like Advocacy VSV stepped in to fill some of the gaps. Niamh Quinn was instrumental in setting up the charity and offering practical and emotional support. Without Niamh's guidance, I might never have made it past the final hurdle in my decision-making.

---

14 Gillen, Sir John. "Northern Ireland Rape Case Review." *The Guardian*, 20 November 2018, https://www.theguardian.com/uk-news/2018/nov/20/northern-ireland-rape-case-review-sir-john-gillen.

15 Northern Ireland Executive. Gillen Review Report: The Law and Procedures in Serious Sexual Offences in Northern Ireland. 2019, https://www.justice-ni.gov.uk/publications/gillen-review-report-law-and-procedures-serious-sexual-offences-ni.

She gave me the kind of safety I'd only ever felt with David. She encouraged me to trust my intuition. Despite the overwhelming odds that justice might not come, my gut told me I needed to report the crime. If I didn't, I'd always be burdened with *what ifs – should I, would I, could I?*

The conflicting voices – mother, sister, daughter, professional – filled my mind with noise. But the autistic part of me cut through it. I relied on my clear, black-and-white thinking, focusing on the facts. Niamh helped me quiet the rest. A crime had been committed. It needed to be reported.

Taking Action

Chapter 43: Truth at the Door, Child at the Gate

I called 101 and reported the rape to the Police Service of Northern Ireland (PSNI) in 2023, just days after meeting Niamh. Naively, I thought I could go back to work after the call. But my body had other plans. I began shaking internally, chilled to the bone, as though the rape had just happened. Overwhelming sensations flooded me.

The passage of time means little to trauma – something the criminal justice system, and many others, fail to understand.

That afternoon, two armed, uniformed male police officers arrived at my home. They were there to gather evidence from the witness of a non-recent rape – an event that had occurred seventeen years ago, but felt as fresh as yesterday. My trauma had frozen me in time.

I will never forget that day. The police recorded a lengthy statement at my home. My six-year-old son arrived home just after the recording and was greeted by the officers. Seeing my child walk in and be confronted by the reality of a police presence jolted me into awareness. I had responsibilities far greater than reporting the rape.

Without Niamh's support, I might have retracted my statement right then. The thought of continuing this process without help for myself and my small family felt impossible.

In the days that followed, I received calls from the rape crime unit to arrange an official ABE (Achieving Best Evidence) interview. I was introduced to the investigating officer who would head the case. I became jumpy, bracing for the next call, never knowing when or who it would be, or what they would say or ask. These weren't the kinds of conversations you want to have while grabbing a loaf of bread or trying to coax your son to do his homework.

The ABE interview was scheduled for early August at the Portadown Rape Crime Unit. Niamh reassured me that she would be with me, both to and from the interview, offering her unwavering support.

Chapter 44: White Trainers on Black Tarmac

As we approached Portadown Police Station, the cold, imposing green steel barricades loomed ahead – an unnervingly stark welcome. They reminded me, in a way, of the Swiss Alps that greeted us when we first arrived in that country: equally imposing, but without the serene beauty. These fences felt like the emotional, mental, and practical obstacles I was facing as a victim. If only the station had the welcoming feel of a cosy community police office – maybe I could have felt more at ease. But instead, it felt like I was driving towards a battlefield, preparing for yet another fight, though I was exhausted from the war I'd already been waging every day.

My thoughts churned as we drew up in the visitor car park. Though I knew I shouldn't worry, I couldn't help but wonder about the investigating officer heading my case. Was she Protestant? As a Catholic, would that cause issues? These concerns, though seemingly trivial, stemmed from the deep-rooted biases of Northern Ireland – biases that linger despite the peace process. I worried my background might influence the proceedings, even down to how I spoke, as pronunciation here can reveal religious affiliation. I thought of the incident after the rape, when the perpetrator paraded me around, pretending we were going to Mass, only to mock me and say we weren't. Should I mention this? Would using the word "Mass" instead of "church" cause complications? Was it even relevant?

My thoughts spiralled, but deep down I knew these concerns, though real, were mostly noise. They weren't the true focus of this moment. As Niamh parked the car and turned off the engine, my mind snapped back to the task at hand.

I opened the car door, and as my white trainers touched the tarmac, I felt a strange detachment. Was this really happening? My body moved mechanically, carrying me towards the investigating officer at the gate. She was much shorter than I'd expected, and that height similarity brought a fleeting comfort. I forced a nervous smile as stray strands of grey hair swept across my face.

"One step at a time," I reminded myself.

Watching Niamh lead the way reassured me. Without her, I wouldn't have been able to sign in. Just walking through those doors would have been too much to bear alone.

While Niamh handled the formalities, I found myself unsure of how to address the investigating officer. Was I speaking to a woman, a mother, a colleague, or simply a professional? My only police experience had been the two officers who visited my home. Should I stick to the basic facts – time, place, event – or share the analytical journey that led me here? There was no guide for this. Victims do not get legal representation, and navigating it all, especially as an autistic person, felt like a threat in itself.

The ABE interview was just as draining as the initial recording at my home. A massive weight was lifted when it was over. For a moment, I felt the burden wasn't mine anymore; it belonged to the police now. The investigating officer complimented me on the valuable information I'd provided, but I was too drained to truly absorb her words. I realised every word, gesture, and emotion may be scrutinised – my tone, my body language, my facial expressions. But I had done it. That was what mattered.

I don't know if Niamh fully understood how much her presence meant. With her beside me, I wasn't just a woman fighting for justice; we were fighting together. She wasn't just my advocate; she was my lifeline. And every victim of this crime deserves someone like her. Niamh's unwavering support shouldn't be a luxury; it should be a basic, non-negotiable part of the process.

The journey to and from the police station felt like a brief chapter in a much longer book. Now, the real waiting game began. Days stretched into weeks, weeks into months. Despite trying to move on, the open case lingered. My trauma, only partially processed, still felt raw, seeping into every part of my life. Thoughts, emotions, and memories surfaced unexpectedly. I tried to live normally, but I was still grappling with understanding my trauma and my response to it.

Later, I learned at a closure meeting with the PPS, with my advocate present, that the defendant's police interview had not been video recorded, only audio. My body language, facial expressions, and emotional state were captured on camera; his were not. That felt like yet another imbalance in the process.

.

Rebuilding

Therapy and Growth

Chapter 45: Not the Perfect Victim—Still Deserving

I had come this far. I had called 101, completed my ABE, and started therapy. I took my medication when needed, and I explored non-conventional healing. I was trying to improve my life. For a while, things seemed to settle. When the ABE was finally over, I felt a wave of relief – but it didn't last. As time passed and the silence from the police and prosecution grew, anxiety crept back.

What's happening? What are they doing? Is no news good news? What is "good" news anyway? Was it when the evidence test fails and the case gets closed? Or when he's charged and goes to trial? To me, there was no clear good or bad outcome. If the case were closed, I could at least say I'd done all I could and try to move on, though disappointed. But after everything, didn't I deserve some semblance of justice?

I tried imagining court, clinging to hope through other survivors' stories, but they were discouraging. I knew I could end up facing the defence team alone, autistic and traumatised, while skilled barristers relentlessly tore at my words, live before a jury. There was no support for that – nothing to protect victims from such ruthless legal bullying.

I thought of Ellie Wilson in Glasgow, who spoke out about her brutal court experience and challenged the defence barrister who bullied her in court.[16] Her bravery should be a wake-up call. But

---

16 BBC News. "Rape Victims' Voices Not Being Heard, Campaigners Say." BBC News, https://www.bbc.co.uk/news/articles/c4n1l3n8zg1o.

in "he-said, she-said" cases, without corroboration, the defendant's word too often holds more weight.

Jade Blue McCrossen-Nethercott's case is an example of this.[17] The prosecution dropped her case right before it was set to go to trial, citing an episode of sexsomnia as evidence it wasn't rape, only to reverse the decision after Jade fought back. The harsh reality hit: without corroborating evidence, a case likely wouldn't make it to court. I wondered – did I have enough? Would my friend make their statement? Was I the kind of victim the prosecution felt confident putting before a jury? I can almost hear the defence planting seeds of doubt: *"She didn't shout for help." "She waited almost two decades – perhaps her memories are flawed."* And if my case went to trial, was I ready? Ready for the barristers to twist my words, confuse me, discredit me? The more I read, the clearer it became: the defence plays a game, hoping victims break under pressure.

Amanda Brown from Northern Ireland described in *No Peace Until He's Dead* how the defence barrister wouldn't even look at her, directing questions to the jury, dehumanising her to sow doubt. The prosecution doesn't know the victim; they represent the Crown, not the person. The burden of proof rests with the prosecution, but in practice, it's the victim who is scrutinised.

I couldn't understand why this was still allowed in today's world. Yes, victims can now testify behind screens or via video link, but that doesn't stop experienced defence lawyers twisting every word. This sort of bullying should be made illegal.

Ellie Wilson's fight to give Scottish victims free access to court notes offered hope. And in her case, the barrister who bullied her

---

17 Topping, A. (2022, October 5). *Woman sues CPS after rape case dropped when man claimed 'sexsomnia'.* The Guardian. https://www.theguardian.com/society/2022/oct/05/jade-mccrossen-nethercott-sue-cps-rape-case-dropped-sexsomnia.

was fined £2,000.[18,19] Small victories, but reminders that change is possible.

Still, one of the biggest barriers isn't just the system – it's society itself. Juries, unequipped to understand trauma, may not grasp how it shapes memory and testimony. Nervousness or imperfect recall gets twisted into unreliability. Amanda Brown said, *"Think about how long it takes us to admit it happened in the first place, think about how long it takes us to sit for hours in the offices of therapists and psychiatrists; how many times we opt for suicide over exposure."*[20] I think of my own case – how long it took me to acknowledge what happened before I could report it. And I wonder how my neurodivergence complicates everything. The system doesn't just fail me – it often doesn't even understand me.[21]

I'm not the perfect victim.

The silence from the PPS gnawed at me. Was I believed? Or would the weight of the defence's words drown out my truth? Despite everything, I take solace in knowing I reported the crime. The allegation is now on his record – it could help support any future allegations.

---

18 BBC News. "Rape Victims' Voices Not Being Heard, Campaigners Say." BBC News, https://www.bbc.co.uk/news/articles/cn3n3ddlmkgo.

19 Edinburgh Live. "Edinburgh Lawyer Fined for 'Unacceptable' Questioning of Rape Survivor." Edinburgh Live, 2022, https://www.edinburghlive.co.uk/news/edinburgh-news/edinburgh-lawyer-fined-over-unacceptable-29197311.

20 Brown, Amanda. *No Peace Until He's Dead.* Merrion Press, 23 February 2024.

21 Fricker, Miranda. "Adopting Fricker's Framework of Testimonial Injustice: The Experiences of Sexual Violence Survivors with Learning Disabilities/Autism." *Disability & Society*, vol. 38, no. 1, 2024, https://www.tandfonline.com/doi/abs/10.1080/09687599.2024.2323455.

And I draw strength from other victims like Haileigh Lamont and Amanda Brown. They don't know me, but their bravery helped me find my voice.[22,23]

And even now, after telling the truth, there is still more to uncover. The analysis continues.

22 *Belfast Telegraph*. "'I Am Victorious': Brave Woman Watches Step-Dad Tommy Harris Jailed After 'Vile' Attacks." *Belfast Telegraph*, https://www.belfasttelegraph.co.uk/news/courts/i-am-victorious-brave-woman-watches-step-dad-tommy-harris-jailed-after-vile-depraved-attacks/41022364.html.

23 "No Peace Until He's Dead." Instagram, https://www.instagram.com/no_peace_until_hes_dead/.

Chapter 46: Pre-Shrunk and Still Growing

As part of the natural progression in my therapeutic journey, I navigated a whirlwind of emotions. When I reached the anger stage – when the full impact of the rape truly landed – I began considering whether or not to report it. It was an agonising decision that took time, energy, and research. I wanted to be informed.

In that process, I reached out to a few organisations that support victims of sexualised crime for confidential advice, and I found myself placed on the waiting list for counselling at Nexus, a charity specialising in treating victims of sexualised violence.

The original plan was to attend a few sessions to help guide my decision about reporting. I hadn't anticipated that the waiting list might stretch into several months, but I understood how high the demand for specialist services like theirs could be. As days turned into weeks, and weeks into months, the weight of knowing that a crime had been committed – one that had derailed my life – and remained unreported became too heavy to carry.

Eventually, without having received any counselling from Nexus, I made the decision to report the rape.

By the time they contacted me with an offer of counselling, I had almost forgotten I was still on their waiting list. I suddenly found myself in a difficult position with my current therapy. Should I stay, or should I go?

After some reflection, I realised there were two compelling reasons to give Nexus a try. First, supporting survivors of sexualised violence is their core focus – it's their bread and butter – and they have a huge reputation. Second, I couldn't help but wonder whether, if my case ever reached court, a jury might question why

I hadn't engaged with a specialist charity like Nexus. That concern lingered in my mind, whether valid or not.

The decision to take a break from my sessions with David wasn't easy. We had built a strong therapeutic alliance, and the thought of stepping away from that felt daunting. I dreaded the conversation. But as always, sitting across from him made it easier. I shared my decision and explained my reasons. He received it with kindness and professionalism, offering his full support as I moved into this next phase of healing. Even in that difficult moment of transition, I felt held, seen, and respected.

Soon after, I found myself sitting across from a new therapist, Fiona.

I'm shown into a quiet consultation room by a warm, open-looking woman with curly brown hair. She smiles as we enter, and I find myself trying to place her age — somewhere between mine and my mother's, perhaps. It doesn't really matter, but I notice myself noting it anyway. There's a calmness in the space. That helps.

She introduces herself as Fiona, and I take a seat opposite her. Her tone is friendly but grounded, her manner easy and present, not forced.

"So," she says gently, "would you like to start by telling me a bit about yourself?"

I've been here before; I know the drill. I nod and smile slightly.

"Sure. I'm Anna. And... I guess you could say I'm 'pre-shrunk'," I half-laugh.

Fiona looks momentarily puzzled, so I explain, "I've done quite a bit of psychoanalysis, ya'no, I've seen a shrink, so I'm not new to therapy, I'm pre-shrunk."

I give a small laugh. She laughs too, and breaks the ice.

My shoulders drop a little. I feel myself settle.

"I'm a mother and a wife. I used to work as a pharmacist. My mum died not that long ago." I pause, then continue, more quietly. "And, you know, I'm…" I stutter slightly. "I'm a rape victim." But I know she knows that already; otherwise, I wouldn't be here.

There's a brief silence – held, not empty. Fiona nods gently.

"Thank you for sharing that."

She then explains how she works: integrative, with lots of psychoeducation. As she talks, I feel myself relax a bit more. It feels supportive, not intrusive.

I let out a little sigh of relief as the anxiety and tension from preparing to be here today started to leave my body.

***

In the sessions that followed, Fiona helped me lay a strong foundation for grounding myself, for feeling safe and returning to the present when my mind defaulted to the past, dragging me back into terror.

Her gentle invitations to speak about the days and weeks after the rape brought back memories I thought were locked away forever. Viewing those events from a distance allowed me to understand not only the rape itself, but also the manipulative games he played afterwards.

I came to see that I wasn't just a victim of rape, but also of manipulation, exploitation, abuse, and dehumanisation. Fiona helped me reflect on how I'd viewed the rapist at the time, and how I could begin to shift that perspective.

He was no longer in control of me.

While much of the work we did together was grounding exer-
cises, I still continued some analysis on my own. As our sessions
continued, in my mind's eye, the image of him grew smaller,
while I grew bigger.

Chapter 47: The Weight of Belief

Fourteen consecutive years of my life were spent in all-girls Catholic schools. For the most part, they were good schools. The teachers and staff were friendly and professional, the education was strong, and there was a real sense of community.

But as institutions under the umbrella of the Catholic Church, no school could escape certain doctrines and indoctrinations, no matter how modern, outspoken, or compassionate the teachers.

Sex education was strictly framed within a religious context, except for the occasional biological lesson covering reproduction. The core message was clear: sex belonged only within marriage, and solely for procreation. Anything else was sinful. The burden of upholding this moral standard fell squarely on us girls, not on any future partners we might have.

There was an unspoken atmosphere of shame woven through it all. "Self-respect" was a term they used constantly. Everything was tied to it. God forbid you didn't have it. Shame was often the tool they used to enforce it.

"Inappropriate" behaviour was strictly defined, from skirt length to necklines. We were regularly reminded of the state of our uniforms.

These teachings left a mark. I developed a quiet shame about my changing body. While many of my peers proudly packed bikinis for summer holidays, I wouldn't be caught dead in one. I preferred full coverage at the beach.

I took the rules seriously, almost literally. I wanted to avoid the sting of shame, the whispers, the labels given to girls who strayed from the path. And it wasn't just about clothes. At age eleven, I took a pledge to abstain from alcohol until I was eighteen. Most of us did. Only a few kept it.

As I moved further into my teens, a natural rebellious streak emerged. I began testing boundaries – wearing outfits that pushed the limits of what the nuns deemed "respectful". There was no malice behind it. It didn't mean I lacked self-respect. I was simply trying to fit in, influenced by the world beyond the school gates. Still, that shame lingered – something I'd only come to understand much later in counselling. Exploring those beliefs in therapy helped me make sense of my nineteen-year-old self, the young woman who was taken by an evil force one night. Traumatised, unable to process what had happened, she carried the shame and responsibility that had been instilled in her, even though she was the victim of something completely beyond her control.

It also helped me understand my friend – the one I confided in less than twelve hours after the assault. Their words still ring in my ears, words that somehow implied I must have invited what happened. Now, I can look back on those days and weeks with new awareness and distance. I see a young woman trying to rationalise what happened, searching for meaning to ease the burden of shame. She convinced herself that maybe he'd fallen in love with her at first sight, that what happened was some twisted "moment of passion".

It was a warped narrative, but one that made the trauma more bearable. A coping mechanism. A way to survive the tsunami that had hit her.

Now, I feel sick thinking how I once equated rape with love. But in hindsight, it's not surprising. I'd been taught that intimacy was sacred, reserved for loving, committed relationships. Anything else, even something violently forced, was incomprehensible.

My Catholic upbringing, my autistic way of processing the world, and my trauma responses worked together to protect me from the horror of what had truly occurred. But they also left me vulnerable. They made me see the best in everyone – even in the man who violated me.

In those weeks, I searched desperately for some shred of goodness in him. He knew exactly what he was doing. He zoned in on my vulnerabilities in that moment of terror. He knew which buttons to press, how to manipulate. He showed up at my halls of residence, spinning stories about how his mother had kicked him out, how he had nowhere to stay. He preyed on my compassion. The belief that he loved me faded after a few weeks. The shame didn't.

For seventeen long years, I blamed myself. I carried that shame until I opened up in the safety of psychotherapy and finally confronted the truth.

I hadn't asked to be raped. I hadn't done anything wrong.

This is part of why I revisited the assault seventeen years later – to finally say those words and believe them.

Now, I often wonder, if we'd been taught about consent, would I have recognised the rape for what it was? If I'd been told my body was mine, that no one had the right to violate it under any circumstances, would I have spoken up sooner?

I hope things have changed in schools today. I think they have.

Education is everything. Be careful what you teach your children. They might just believe every word.

Chapter 48: Taking the Wheel

For years, when getting behind the wheel was necessary to move from A to B, I simply didn't go. This avoidance began shortly after I passed my driving test in February 2007, but I could never pinpoint why fear had suddenly taken hold.

Therapy brought about change. And after nearly fourteen years of restricting myself to the passenger seat, driving became one of those changes.

Being dependent on others and public transport impacted my life in ways I hadn't fully realised. My career, social life, and ability to carry out daily tasks all suffered, and my self-confidence took a huge hit. Despite this, I never considered my inability to drive as a disability, nor did I recognise it as a trauma response. Much like how I couldn't bring myself to call what happened to me "rape", I couldn't associate my driving issues with disability. I had never thought of myself that way. After all, labelling myself as "disabled" would mean facing up to something broken in my life – something I was still trying to avoid.

But the truth was: I was living with a disability. I had PTSD. Rationalising it away, invalidating my experiences – this had become my way of coping, just as it had with the trauma of rape.

My family offered lifts, and when I met Marek, he unwittingly stepped into a caring role, filling the gaps. Living in Switzerland helped too. The country's impeccable public transport system allowed me to blend in, relying on trains and buses instead of confronting my fear of driving.

Returning to the wheel was a slow, gradual process. Routine trips that most people take for granted required an overwhelming amount of mental energy. I had to psyche myself up before each journey, consciously keeping calm while navigating everyday tasks. With Marek by my side – taking on more than most husbands and fathers do – I was spared much of the distress.

But on one particular November day in 2023, I had to collect my son from school while Marek was busy with work. It was a familiar journey, one I'd done countless times as a passenger, and even as a driver. But it still took significant effort to stay calm.

As I ascended the familiar hill, the vibrant colours of autumn surrounded me. A lone leaf drifted from the kerbside, landing squarely in my path. I saw it move from the corner of my eye, already predicting it would drift into my car's path. But even though I anticipated it, my body reacted as if I hadn't. My heart leapt. My foot slammed towards the brake pedal. Then, mid-action, I stopped myself. It was only a leaf.

In those few seconds, I realised my body lived in a state of constant readiness – perpetually alert, waiting to fight or flee. Thankfully, my logical brain kicked in and whispered, "*Anna, it's only a leaf*," and with that, I eased off the brake.

Now that I understand how hypervigilance affects my driving, I can also see how it seeps into other parts of my life. Simple tasks often require an exhausting amount of effort, and I sometimes react excessively. This hypervigilance is PTSD. It has drained me for years, flying under the radar, undiagnosed.

People with PTSD are often like leaves blowing in the wind – unseen by others who haven't experienced trauma, or haven't processed their own. We feel alone in our daily battles, swayed by life's unpredictable gusts. And yet, I've had to acknowledge my resilience. Even with these challenges, I've managed to push through everyday tasks that others take for granted. But that same resilience has also held me back. I could have had the right support, and I might have avoided being so constantly drained. To truly move forward, I needed to accept my limitations.

Getting from A to B is an achievement in itself, both literally and metaphorically. And if I cannot make it to C, I need to accept that too, instead of fighting it. Acceptance is part of healing. I'll never be the person I was before the trauma of 2006. Coming to terms with this feels like mourning the life I thought I would have.

Like the leaf I saw blowing in the wind that day, I was once tossed around by life's forces, lacking control. But "was" is the key word. I now *choose* to drive my own car. And with the right support, I can.

Chapter 49: Invisible Fault Lines

Describing the change that happens in someone after rape is incredibly difficult. Rape is a distinct and devastating crime, leaving behind a unique kind of trauma. I didn't fully understand the extent of the changes in myself until I began to process what had happened. Only then did I start to see things for what they truly were.

Before that, I had created an illusion for myself and for those around me. It was a survival mechanism, one that helped me function, helped me complete my university degree. At the time, it felt like an achievement, a way to regain some control. But looking back, I can see that getting that degree was the least of my concerns.

I wish I had allowed myself to pause, to take time out and deal with what had happened. If I had, maybe I could have reclaimed a sense of agency, made choices rooted in my needs, and started living more authentically.

Now, nearly two decades later, I'm facing the painful truth that I haven't been my true self for most of my adult life – and even much of my childhood. I'm still not entirely sure who that authentic self is, but through therapy, I'm starting to uncover her. She's slowly beginning to find her voice.

There are no words in the dictionary that fully capture the overwhelming fear that follows a traumatic experience like rape. It disrupted everything: my body, my mind, my thoughts, my emotions. Fear became a default setting – so deeply embedded that it began to feel like part of my identity. It made trusting others nearly impossible, even those closest to me. I began to see the world as a dark, dangerous place, filled with people I could not rely on.

And if you do not know who you are, how can you build real relationships? Without understanding and accepting yourself, how can others connect with you? These questions haunt me when I think about every relationship I've had – friends, family, romantic partners, colleagues.

After the assault, I lived behind the illusion I'd constructed. I withdrew from my social circle and distanced myself from friends. Even family relationships became strained, despite my efforts to maintain them. Trauma responses – so misunderstood and often invisible – created a gulf between me and the people I cared about.

Making friends has always been difficult for me. The bond I thought I had with *a friend* – the one I reached out to after the rape – was, I now realise, not what I believed it to be.

Therapy helped me uncover deeper truths about myself, including a late diagnosis of autism. That revelation brought clarity to a lifetime of confusion. I finally understood why I had struggled to connect – why making friends often felt like deciphering a code that others seemed to know instinctively.

And yet, it wasn't always impossible. When I first moved away from home and lived in university halls, I made new connections. Genuine ones. One person in particular, Colleen, stands out in my memory. I remember her with great affection. But after the assault, that connection changed. Everything changed. Belfast didn't feel safe anymore. Newry didn't feel safe. Nowhere felt safe. I began locking doors – both literal and metaphorical. I stopped reaching out. The invitations stopped coming. I slowly disappeared from social life, and eventually, from Colleen too.

Chapter 50: It Started With a Message

As I reflected on the relationships I had before and after the rape, a deep anger surfaced. Someone had stolen my power – my sense of control over my own life. I decided it was time to reclaim it. I began to think about the friendships I had left behind, and one person kept coming to mind: Colleen. The thought of reconnecting with her stirred anxiety. So much time had passed. How could I explain my disappearance? Would she think I was strange? What had her life been like since then? Was she still the same Colleen I remembered?

After some inner debate, I chose to take the risk. What was the worst that could happen – rejection? I'd faced far worse.

So, with a nervous flutter in my chest, I reached out to her through social media. I didn't expect anything. I just wanted to see what might happen.

I sent her a message:

"Hi Colleen, how are you doing? I know this message is out of the blue, it's been such a long time. How are things? I saw you're living in [location] now! That's not far from me."

Then I closed the app and tried to go about my day.

To my surprise, she replied within the hour. We messaged back and forth for the rest of the day, and before long, she invited me to visit. Her warmth, her enthusiasm, her simple appreciation that I had reached out – it was more than I could have hoped for.

When I arrived at her farmhouse in the Cooley Peninsula, a wave of emotion washed over me. Good memories – the ones that had been buried by trauma – came rushing back. Colleen hadn't changed. Her dry humour, her relaxed presence, and that familiar warmth were still there. But her life had moved on. She was now married, pregnant, and living a new chapter. I stood there marvelling at how much had changed for both of us.

She welcomed me back with open arms – literally. Over the course of that visit, she hugged me four times. I wondered if she knew how much those hugs meant to me, or if she was quietly counting them too, like I was.

The second time we met, we had lunch at The Oliver in Newry and spent the afternoon wandering the shopping centre. It felt like time had folded in on itself – like we were back in those carefree days, laughing, chatting, enjoying the ease of each other's company.

Despite the years that had separated us, that special bond reignited. For the first time in what felt like forever, I felt a surge of life return to me. I even noticed something familiar in myself. When we walked into the shopping centre, I felt that familiar pang of anxiety in my stomach. But instead of letting it swallow me, I acknowledged it. I reminded myself I was safe, especially with Colleen beside me. I didn't shrink away. I faced it, and it passed.

In that moment, I felt something I hadn't felt in years: happiness. Not just surface happiness, but the kind that lets you breathe freely. Like you're no longer treading water. Like you've finally found your way back to solid ground.

Since I reached out, Colleen and I have stayed in touch. We meet as often as we can. Our doors – and hearts – are open to one another again. What once felt lost is being rebuilt, one moment at a time.

Identity Revealed

Chapter 51: The Mask Behind the Mask

For those who have endured trauma, sometimes it feels like they do not even recognise themselves in the mirror. I am one of those people.

Looking into the metaphorical mirror, as in psychoanalysis, was no different. Week after week, I dissected fragments of my being. Some parts I hadn't even been aware of. The discovery of these pieces was often shocking. Sometimes, a breakthrough. Sometimes, just a gateway to more therapy.

Other parts, however, I already knew.

During therapy, certain common themes emerged. These weren't only tied to my trauma; they were intricately connected to my own personality. Obsessive traits became apparent, like my tendency to immerse myself in special interests, spending countless hours on projects before dropping them and moving on. After significant events in my life, this behaviour intensified. I'd fixate entirely on one project, unable to focus on anything else.

This tendency only grew after traumatic experiences – particularly after the night I was raped, and again after my mum's death.

My therapeutic journey unfolded in parallel with another journey – one with my son.

Eventually diagnosed as autistic, he opened a new lens through which I began to question my own neurodiversity.

When I mention the possibility of my own autism to David, he smiles gently and nods, as though he already knows.

There's no formal diagnosis, but he doesn't dismiss the possibility either. His tone is thoughtful, steady, as he points out the striking similarities between my autistic son and me.

I feel the words settle in my chest like pebbles dropping into still water – small ripples, quiet but persistent.

***

Some months later, I met the attuned Fiona at Nexus.

Her voice is warm but direct when she asks, "Anna, have you ever considered getting assessed for neurodiversity?"

I pause, then smile and nod back, a flicker of relief and recognition rising in my body.

"Actually, yes. I've already put myself on the waiting list," I say, trying to moderate the slight enthusiasm that's rising with my voice.

Her laptop, on the other side of the therapy room, gives off a low hum as the fan kicks in. I notice the soft scratch of my fingers as they dig into my jeans, as though trying to anchor myself.

Though I've been questioning my neurodiversity for a while, part of me still clings to denial, like a fog that hasn't quite lifted.

***

Chapter 52: It Cannot Be Me

I could not accept that I was autistic. How could I possibly be autistic and get this far in life without knowing? I had scheduled an appointment with a psychiatrist, believing my symptoms were tied to obsessive-compulsive disorder (OCD) as part of my PTSD, rather than autism. It made more sense to me, especially my irrational fear of driving, convinced I might harm myself or others on the road – an OCD-related trait.

But within just 30 minutes of meeting the psychiatrist, he picked up on my unusual traits. He gave me a questionnaire about my responses, emotions, and thoughts in specific scenarios. My score was exceptionally high, indicating strong autistic traits. After further discussion, he suggested I quietly consider myself autistic and move forward with therapy under that assumption. He also referred me to the NHS for an autism and ADHD assessment, as I had scored highly for ADHD as well.

I wasn't entirely sure about being autistic, but it would explain so much about my childhood. While reading more on the topic, I came across an article claiming that nine out of ten autistic women had been victims of sexualised violence.[24] Though the research was limited, that headline struck me deeply. Had my autism made me more vulnerable to predators? Or was I assaulted because of it?

The search for answers continues. If I am autistic, it means I've been masking over a mask. And until I received an official diagnosis, I felt uneasy about my therapeutic journey.

---

24 Cazalis, F., Reyes, E., Leduc, S., and Gourion, D. "Evidence That Nine Autistic Women Out of Ten Have Been Victims of Sexual Violence." *Frontiers in Behavioral Neuroscience*, vol. 16, 26 April 2022, article 852203. https://doi.org/10.3389/fnbeh.2022.852203.

Chapter 53: Naming What Was Always There

On one cold February afternoon in 2024, my nerves tighten, squeezing my chest with a heavy, anxious weight. I hesitate for a moment before asking the psychologist, "Do you think I am autistic?" The words escape in a rush, as if my heart has beaten them out of me. My mind blurs with questions and doubts as I anxiously wait for her response.

What if she doesn't validate it? What if this entire search for clarity has been in vain? What if she says no, and I have to begin again, searching for who I truly am? But if she says yes... How will I process that? Worse still, what if she leaves me hanging over the weekend?

Then, almost as if reading my thoughts, she says simply, "Yes, you are autistic. You're scoring quite high according to the DSM-5." The words hit me with a strange mixture of relief and emotional overwhelm. My breath catches, and my vision blurs with tears. I tell myself to "wise up". I need to focus. I need to get to the end of this assessment. Crying will only drag it out.

***

As the assessment ends, I slam my laptop shut and sit in a thick fog. I have no one to talk to about this revelation. Marek is caught up in back-to-back meetings, and the only person I truly want to share this with – my mum – is gone. My dad and Toodles are in Australia, and coordinating a call will only make me feel more alone.

I think about calling Cuddles, but she is deep in the throes of new motherhood. I feel guilty for burdening her with my news.

Reluctantly, I pick up the phone and dial. My voice is tight as I share my diagnosis. Cuddles responds with a calmness that surprises me, almost as if she's known this all along. No surprise. No shock. Just a quiet acknowledgment.

I end the call quickly, not wanting to take up too much of her time. Sitting on my bed, I stare at the walls, the silence pressing in around me. What am I supposed to make of this?

Though I've anticipated something like this, especially after everything I've learned through my son's autism assessment, hearing the official diagnosis shakes me more than I expect. It feels like a new layer of self has been unearthed, one that has always been just beneath the surface.

I've spent two years in therapy, coming to terms with my C-PTSD and unpacking the traumas that led to it. I thought I was peeling away the mask of childhood trauma, only to find another mask underneath: autism. It's as though I've been wearing two masks all along. One to conceal my autism. The other to hide the trauma that has shaped my life.

It hit me like a blow. Like unwrapping a present only to find more wrapping underneath.

Who the hell am I? The question echoes in my head, threatening to drown me in a sea of confusion.

Was I ever truly me?

Integration

Chapter 54: What Lies Beneath

After my autism diagnosis, an internal war broke out. I questioned everything. Maybe my son wasn't autistic after all – maybe he was just mimicking me. Doubt crept in, making me wonder whether psychologists truly understood anything at all. Perhaps autism was just another way of describing the messy variety of human experience. Maybe it was just a label –a convenience.

I spiralled into a rabbit hole of questions: What does autism actually mean? Is it just a trendy term people are throwing around on Instagram? I didn't want to latch onto a trend. This wasn't about that. It was about discovering myself – understanding who I really was beneath all the masks and expectations.

As I began yet another journey of self-exploration, I saw clearly how deeply I'd conformed to what others expected of me. I had thought I was reaching the end of my psychoanalytic journey. But the truth was, I had only just scratched the surface. There was still another mask left to peel away. The work was far from over.

Chapter 55: Laughter Before the Grief

Now I wondered if my autism was the reason I had always felt different, and whether that difference made me more vulnerable. If the predator had been able to pick up on my vulnerabilities that night, in a room full of neurotypical women, it made me wonder: Who else had seen it? If it was so obvious to him, why hadn't anyone else seen it? Why hadn't my parents, my teachers, or the adults around me recognised the signs?

But maybe some people had. People who didn't have my best interests at heart. And I wasn't ready to face that – at least, not yet. A familiar feeling of neglect crept in, but I knew it wasn't that simple. I had been an almost perfect masker. How could they have known?

In one of my recent therapy sessions with David, something clicked. He helps me see the roles that have been assigned to me in my family – roles I hadn't fully understood until now. It feels as though I've been exposed in a way that is painful to acknowledge. The realisation lands so sharply, so deeply, that I start laughing. But the laughter quickly gives way to tears. And for a moment, I am laughing and crying at the same time.

I haven't yet received my formal autism diagnosis, but I can feel it coming. The pieces are falling into place.

***

The psychologist who assessed me, with little knowledge of my psychoanalytic journey, mentioned how often autistic children are blamed for everything. As soon as she said it, I knew exactly what she meant. It was like turning a key in a lock – the final piece falling into place. The scapegoat role, as David had described, now made complete sense.

In just two weeks, my understanding of myself and my past shifted profoundly. It was as if the jigsaw puzzle I'd been trying to piece together my entire life had finally started to reveal its image.

And just when I thought psychoanalysis was bringing me clarity, I sensed that this breakthrough was likely the calm before the storm. I'd been here before. When I first realised I had PTSD, the weight of it had sent me spiralling – relapsing into depression, and making choices that had disastrous consequences, like meeting up with the man who raped me.

Should I mentally prepare myself for the storm ahead? Should I brace for another round of emotional chaos?

Sometimes when I try to explain this journey to others, it feels like they don't truly understand what it means. The magnitude of it is lost on them. I don't know if I've learned enough from the past to avoid making the same mistakes, but I write all of this down in the hope that I have. I write in search of clarity, even if I fear my story might be too heavy for others to carry.

Chapter 56: Channelling Anger

By my eighth session with Fiona, I begin to open up about the days and weeks that followed the life-altering event. As the words leave my mouth for the first time, something shifts inside me. A cold, creeping awareness begins to settle – one that stretches far beyond my own naivety or the event itself.

I see it now, in painful clarity: the same person who hurt me didn't just do it once. The abuse, the manipulation, it stretches on, threaded through time far longer than I had allowed myself to acknowledge. His actions weren't impulsive or drunken mistakes. They were deliberate. Planned. Every move – from the violation to his behaviour afterwards – was calculated.

Even the gestures I once mistook for affection, for concern, were exposed for what they really were: hollow, manipulative, designed only to protect himself.

The room around me feels still, yet heavy. Fiona sits quietly across from me, giving the realisation room to breathe. My chest tightens. I grip the sides of my chair. The truth stings   sharp and dizzying – but it's also a beginning.

***

At the time, I couldn't act on my intuition. He had stripped me of all power and control. I had never encountered such deceit, such evil. Or had I? Maybe it was all too familiar?

His sneakiness was immeasurable. And yet, the betrayal I felt from a friend was even more devastating than what I had endured at his hands – but more on that later.

This man didn't just harm me physically, mentally, and emotionally. He destroyed my self-worth. Crushed my confidence. Stole

149

my independence. Once he was done, he discarded me – and with it, my remaining trust in humanity. He controlled not just my body, but my reality. He constructed a narrative. A defence. One so carefully built it could survive scrutiny, even in court. His efforts to appear publicly with me in the days and weeks following the first violation were, in many ways, even more shocking than the assault itself. It was as if he had done this before.

My intuition screamed that I wasn't his only victim.

And then it hit me – I had been vulnerable to manipulative characters like him before. This wasn't the first time I had suffered mental and emotional abuse. And the hardest truth? It wasn't the first time I'd experienced sexual abuse either.

When that memory surfaced, I let it go. It was too much. Not now. Maybe not ever.

What this man did to me had a profound effect. He flooded me with fear, manipulated me emotionally, and, in doing so, awakened other buried trauma.

In this therapy session with Fiona, I have an epiphany. I realise the trauma he caused is one huge, dirty root of my deep self-doubt as an adult. He targeted me at a pivotal time in my life, just as I was stepping into adulthood, beginning university. Not only did he create an illusion for others that we were in a relationship, but he painted that illusion for me too. It was like brushing a vibrant colour over a dark, painful image, the truth buried beneath, hidden too long. I've always known it, somewhere deep down, but I hadn't been ready to confront it, until now.

Now I see it for what it was.

My anger has sharpened. It no longer simmers quietly – it burns. But this time, I don't drown it in alcohol. I sit with it. I let it crackle through me. I give it purpose. It fuels this book. It fuels my commit-

ment to seek justice. My anger needs a visible outlet. The power of an angry woman is something no man can ignore.

Maybe my anger will surprise people, especially in a world that teaches girls to bury their fury, to label it hysteria or hormones. But I stand firm in it.

And as I write, I discover something else: not all of this anger belongs to me. Some of it belongs to him. Emotions, like energy, don't disappear. They move. If they're blocked, they fester.

He carries rage – and he unleashed it on me when he raped me.

I wonder what made him so angry. Where did that darkness come from? No one is born evil. Who taught him this?

Now, I understand how my own buried anger has shaped my life, led me into years of self-destructive patterns, stress-related illnesses, and a fractured sense of self. The clarity hurts, but it's necessary.

I worry about my health, what it's done to my body. But more than that, I worry how this unspoken rage might ripple into my son's life. Children reflect what they see.

I refuse to let him inherit my wounds.

***

Chapter 57: Fault with Forgiveness

In my naivety, I thought I would find the answers I needed when I met with the rapist in the hotel. The air had a chill to it that day, but the encounter itself felt colder, heavier, like a weight pressing on my chest. I had hoped that confronting him would grant me the clarity I longed for: a sense of closure, a chance to ask the questions that had haunted me for years. But that meeting left me empty. I couldn't find the words to express how deeply the rape had affected me, and my questions went unanswered. The failure of what I'd hoped would be restorative justice – even if informal – left me with the same gnawing uncertainty I'd had before. The disappointment lingered long after, like a persistent shadow that wouldn't fade.

By 2024, I'm not sure I've fully recovered from that day. Since then, I've unravelled more about myself – about the way I've allowed others to treat me, and the harsh reality of certain "close" relationships in my life. One of the most painful revelations came in spring 2024, after a final betrayal from one of my friends. The blow was harsh and damaging, like an emotional wound reopening, raw and fresh. That betrayal pushed me deeper into self-reflection, forcing me to face some uncomfortable truths about why I'd been so vulnerable to abuse. What I discovered was a lesson I never wanted to learn: my tendency to "turn a blind eye", and – above all – my endless capacity for forgiveness.

I'd unknowingly given people a free pass to hurt me through my naive and forgiving nature. I'd convinced myself that forgiveness was the key to moving on – even when it came to forgiving the man who raped me. It was as though I was offering absolution as a way of dealing with my trauma. But that forgiveness came at a cost I hadn't fully understood. The more I examined it, the more I realised how deep my vulnerability ran – how I'd been conditioned to accept disrespect and abuse, to forgive and move on as though it were normal.

The realisation hit hard.

I can now see why forgiveness isn't possible for many victims – and how even the idea of it could feel deeply disturbing. I used to believe that my willingness to forgive was part of healing. But through my experiences in 2024, I've come to understand that forgiveness, for me, wasn't so much healing as a coping mechanism – something I developed after years of turning a blind eye to manipulation, intimidation, and bullying. I was conditioned to let it slide, to be the person who forgives, keeps moving forward as though it didn't hurt. The more I explored this, the more I realised it was likely tied to my friend/fawn trauma response – a reflex I'm only beginning to understand.

My childhood conditioning is something I know I need to unpack more in therapy, though it's hard. I still resist diving deeper, mainly because I know how painful it will be. There's only so much emotional weight I can carry at once.

I've come to understand that while forgiveness is often seen as noble, it's also misunderstood. Some people interpret it as a weakness. From my own experience, I now see the trouble with forgiveness as a three-fold. First, psychopaths and narcissists can exploit the forgiving nature to continue abusing. Second, forgiveness can be seen as absolving the perpetrator of their guilt. Third, it can become a distraction, taking focus away from the victim's healing. It's okay to be angry. It's okay to want your perpetrator to feel pain. Forgiveness should never be an expectation placed on the victim. The perpetrator is not entitled to it – it's a right that lies solely with the victim, a power we can grant or withhold.

Then I wonder about the practicalities of forgiveness in my own case. Sometimes, I think it could bring me peace, a way to move forward. But I also recognise the complications. What if the defence used it against me in court? What if they twisted it to discredit me? If they read that I'd forgiven the man who raped me, could they use that to cast doubt in the jury's mind? It's a thought that gnaws at me, casting shadows over any potential sense of closure.

Healing and Family

Chapter 58: Unconventional Therapies

As part of my journey towards healing, I've read extensively on trauma. Dr Gabor Maté and Bessel van der Kolk are two of my preferred authors. I've also explored mindfulness, drawing inspiration from Eckhart Tolle's writing. In addition, I've studied psychedelic-assisted psychotherapy through books and documentaries, especially those by Michael Pollan. Despite the growing body of research on trauma and its neurological effects, I'm still surprised by how little understanding there is around PTSD among healthcare professionals in primary and secondary care. I hope this changes in time.

There are multiple alternative treatments for PTSD that haven't yet been fully embraced by conventional medical professionals. Often, they're dismissed due to "insufficient evidence of effectiveness", but I wonder if this shuts down important conversations and learning opportunities. Functional doctors, by contrast, tend to take a broader view. They recognise that conventional medicine doesn't always offer complete solutions, especially when it comes to PTSD, or many other conditions.

Some of the more unconventional interventions I've come across show real promise. One is the stellate ganglion block, a neck injection that may reset the fight-or-flight response in just one or two administrations.[25] Combined with psychotherapy, it shows

25 Kirkpatrick, K., et al. "A Review of Stellate Ganglion Block as an Adjunctive Treatment Modality." *Cureus*, vol. 15, no. 2, 19 February 2023, article e35174. https://doi.org/10.7759/cureus.35174.

promise.[26] Another is low-dose naltrexone (LDN) an off-label medication that has shown potential in reducing symptoms associated with trauma, according to some clinicians and anecdotal reports.[27] I'm currently on LDN, and while my symptoms are complex, I've found falling asleep easier, and I no longer feel the same draw towards alcohol to manage stress – something that aligns with LDN's primary indication at higher doses. I can't say how much it helps with my PTSD specifically, but I have noticed other health benefits.

Other innovative treatments I've explored include Neurofeed-back[28] and Transcranial Magnetic Stimulation (TMS)[29]. Both have scientific backing that's worth paying attention to, even if they are still considered experimental. Psychedelic-assisted psychotherapy, in particular, is gaining attention, with new research and private investment driving interest. Access remains limited and highly regulated, but with ongoing global trials and encouraging early results, the potential is there.

While the possibility of completely healing from trauma in 2024 remains uncertain, learning to cope with its consequences is achievable and easing the impact is possible. A multidimensional approach helps. This has become a special interest of mine. This

---

26 Lynch, J.H., et al. "Behavioral Health Clinicians Endorse Stellate Ganglion Block as a Valuable Intervention in the Treatment of Trauma-Related Disorders." *Journal of Investigative Medicine*, vol. 69, no. 5, June 2021, pp. 989–993. https://doi.org/10.1136/jim-2020-001693.

27 LDN Research Trust. https://ldnresearchtrust.org/

28 Chiba, T., et al. "Current Status of Neurofeedback for Post-Traumatic Stress Disorder: A Systematic Review and the Possibility of Decoded Neurofeedback." *Frontiers in Human Neuroscience*, 17 July 2019, article 233. https://doi.org/10.3389/fnhum.2019.00233.

29 Petrosino, N.J., et al. "Transcranial Magnetic Stimulation for Post-Traumatic Stress Disorder." *Therapeutic Advances in Psychopharmacology*, 28 October 2021, article 20451253211049921. https://doi.org/10.1177/20451253211049921.

approach addresses the physical, emotional, and mental aspects of health and works towards balance. Practices like yoga, building genuine connections, spending time with loved ones, counselling, hobbies, meditation, good nutrition, time in nature, and spiritual or creative exploration all contribute. I haven't mastered them all, but I see them as something to strive for.

It's important to recognise that most of these treatments are not endorsed by the conventional medical community and are not always accessible or affordable. If you are considering such treatment for yourself, it's recommended to speak to your GP and only access such treatment from a registered healthcare professional.

When it comes to conventional medicine, I remain cautiously hopeful. I believe meaningful change will only come when our health systems begin to take trauma seriously – when patients are offered a broader range of options, and some control over how they heal. That could make all the difference, especially for those of us who have experienced profound powerlessness.

Chapter 59: Impact on Those Around Me

Rape is catastrophic. It doesn't only affect the victim – it ripples outwards, impacting everyone around them. One day, I was changed, as if a switch had been flipped in my brain. The "Anna" that my parents, siblings, friends, and others once knew was gone. In her place was an empty vessel pretending to be Anna. The authentic relationships I once had disappeared, and every relationship I formed after that was built on trauma.

I remember my dad calling me "Hurricane Anna" when I returned home from university in my third and fourth years. It was a nickname he'd never used before. "Hurricane" replaced my former one: "Petals". My mum watched as I lost a significant amount of weight in a short space of time and suffered panic attacks. Both my parents – and Cuddles – saw me gripped by terror trying to get into a car and drive, often abandoning the journey halfway through. The Anna who had been finding herself, settling into university, exploring new friendships and nurturing old ones, was gone. I stopped socialising. I left my job. A few years later, after I returned from Florence, my mum quietly said to Toodles, "I feel like I've lost my daughter."

As I write this, I'm devastated – because Mum wasn't wrong. And now, she's no longer here for me to explain everything to. The cost of my trauma on those around me is immeasurable. But it didn't just affect those close to me at the time of the rape or in the years that followed. My trauma ripples out still, touching everyone I encounter, even now.

One example stands out. It was March 2023, and my son said something that struck me so deeply, I had to write it down. The conversation went like this:

"Mummy," he called out a few times. I didn't respond. So he asked, "Mummy, why do you do that?"

I finally realised he was speaking to me. "Do what?" I asked.

"Why do you freeze like that?"

"Freeze? What do you mean?"

"You do it a lot," he said. "It's like you go into a different world and leave your body here. When you go into the different world, do you just bring your spirit with you?"

Grief surged through me as I looked at him – my son, with his big, innocent eyes – staring up at me. I tried to explain: "It's because Mummy has adult stress stuck inside her. And when Nanny died, it made it worse. Sometimes the stress makes Mummy go into a different world, but I'm trying to make it better. It will take time."

He thought for a moment. "Okay, why don't we turn off the sun for a whole day and a whole night, so when you wake up, Mummy, you can forget about it?"

I replied, "Wow, that's a very smart idea. Wouldn't it be lovely if we could do that – like recharging ourselves? But unfortunately, we can't. Thank you, son, for sharing your thoughts with me."

I kept thanking him. I'm trying to practise conscious parenting. I want him to feel seen, heard, and validated – because I felt so lacking in those things, and the rape magnified that feeling of invisibility. I explained that it was good that he told me. I asked him to keep reminding me when it happens, because it helps me "wake up".

Since then, I've often heard him say, "Mummy, you're doing it again," or "Mummy, you're freezing again," and sometimes, "Mummy, wake up."

He was only six years old, and yet he had already identified – and verbalised – my dissociation. While I was impressed by his insight, my heart broke. How much had he seen before he had the language to tell me?

Now, I reflect on how my trauma might have influenced my parenting. I do so not from a place of blame, but of growth and understanding. Some research has shown that maternal trauma can impact neurodevelopmental disorders in offspring.[30] While I'm autistic myself, I don't deny the potential effects trauma could have on children. Trauma can profoundly affect human physiology, and the topics of intergenerational trauma and genetics, especially epigenetics, where environment and genetics interact, are vast areas that deserve more open, compassionate exploration.

30 Roberts, A.L., et al. "Women's Posttraumatic Stress Symptoms and Autism Spectrum Disorder in Their Children." *Research in Autism Spectrum Disorders*, vol. 8, no. 6, 1 June 2014, pp. 608–616. https://doi.org/10.1016/j.rasd.2014.02.004.

Dreams and Reflection

Sometimes my dreams speak the truths I still struggle to say out loud.

Chapter 60: Between the Ice and the Iron

In December 2023, I found myself dangling from the balcony rail of a cruise ship, surrounded by women and girls. My knuckles were white as I clung to the rail, caught between two equally terrifying choices: plunge into the freezing Arctic waters below or pull myself back onto the ship. But staying meant returning to a waking nightmare – a vessel ruled by a dangerous man, where women lived trapped under his abusive dominance.

I chose to climb back aboard. My only hope was to manage or change the situation – something I couldn't do if I disappeared into the sea. But once I was back, I realised I was being hunted. He was after me. The ship was his prison, and he was the governor.

As I ran past cabins and communal spaces, I saw women following his orders like obedient shadows. Then I passed a large room filled with women at sewing machines. At first, I thought they were enslaved – but they were secretly preparing to escape, stitching together a plan. They needed strength; they needed protection. I wanted to help them.

I kept running, eventually finding a dark attic-like space on the top deck. Dusty and claustrophobic. There, I discovered a heartbreaking sight: little girls hiding in fear. I knew they couldn't stay there. Time was running out. I had to prepare them, even if it meant forcing them to grow up too soon. I led them out, urging them to stay quiet, keep their heads down, and join the women below.

Then I turned back to face him. I needed to buy time. I tried to stay calm, to befriend him, anything to stall him. But he became aggressive. He pushed me into a narrow corridor and exposed himself. I didn't want this. I tried to fight, but fear paralysed me.

I woke up just as it happened – heart pounding, sick with shame and terror.

Dreams like this have haunted me for seventeen years. I used to think they were just nightmares. Everyone has bad dreams, don't they? But now I know these are trauma flashbacks. In these dreams, I'm always in danger. I'm hunted, silenced, hurt, powerless. I cry for help and no one comes. I curl up alone, afraid. Sometimes I lose my son. Sometimes I'm assaulted again.

Even when life is calm, the dreams return. My subconscious won't let me rest. They remind me that the trauma is still there, festering.

For most of my adult life, I didn't realise they were trauma responses. I thought I was just a poor sleeper. But each night, I relived the assault. The same dread, the same nausea, the same pounding heart. The same wound reopened again and again.

Now I understand – trauma doesn't just live in the memory. It lives in the body. It steals sleep, safety, and peace.

Chapter 61: Left Behind in a Language I Do Not Speak

I was in India – a place I've never been. Crawling through metal tunnels, climbing narrow ladders, squeezing through manholes. The air was thick. My skin was slick with sweat, my breathing shallow. There was something deeply wrong about this place.

Eventually, I reached a presentation room. I was there to meet employees. They proudly unveiled a laser beam product, boasting that it operated above legal frequency limits. Before I could respond, they turned it on. White light flooded the room – intense, invasive. "Don't look directly at it," they warned. "You could go blind."

I panicked. I had to get out. The beams flickered at the edge of my vision like ghosts. Had they already damaged my eyes?

I stumbled through shadowed corridors, heart pounding. I reached a metal escape chute and slid down. Ahead of me were two girls from my old school. I called out. They didn't turn around. They didn't wait. They climbed into a black car with tinted windows. A private driver was waiting. The doors shut. The engine revved. They left.

I stood alone, whispering, "I'm going to Florence too," though no one could hear me. The weight of invisibility pressed in. India felt like a symbol for something else – a place tied to secrecy or danger, where I didn't belong. I wasn't part of their world. I was left behind, again.

I woke up with my face in the pillow, drenched in relief that it had only been a dream. But it was the third in recent weeks – always with the same themes: fear, tunnels, crime, abandonment. This time, the setting was foreign. There was no theft. Just abandonment.

Aftermath

Chapter 62: Surrendering

"You don't have to control your thoughts. You just have to stop letting them control you."

— DAN MILLMAN

Dreams have become a gateway in my therapy with David. When I don't know where to begin, I start with the images that visited me during the night. Since my autism diagnosis, the recurring dreams of falling behind, of being unseen, have begun to make sense.

For years, I've masked who I am. Tried to keep up. Tried to be who the world expected. But in dreams, I am always struggling to catch up, or I'm left behind. Often, I am robbed – a handbag stolen, my voice silenced. And I now see what's really being taken: my identity, my autonomy. That night, at nineteen years of age, didn't just traumatise me – it fractured something essential. My safety. My sense of self.

That predator may have seen something in me – signs of neurodivergence I didn't yet have language for. Autistic women are statistically more likely to be victims of sexual assault. I didn't know that before, but now I do. And I know it matters.

The ladders in my dreams – the climbing, the falling – are metaphors. They reflect my inner journey, my struggle to keep up, to rise, to belong. But maybe the answer isn't to keep trying. Maybe it's to stop pretending.

I'm burned out. I've been performing for years, and I'm tired. The mask I wear is wearing me down. And beneath it, I've become invisible. It's time to let that mask go. But I don't know how.

What saddens me most is how deeply trauma has amplified my autistic challenges. I might never "fit in" – not the way others do. But I don't need to. I can create a different life, one on my terms. I don't have to chase what was never mine.

This will be painful. Letting go always is. But it's time. It's time to surrender – not to despair, but to the truth. To who I really am.

The End of the Case, Not the Story

Chapter 63: A Letter Without Warning

Wednesday at 11 a.m. is always an important time for me. I reserve this hour for my weekly psychotherapy session, and no matter what else is happening in my life, I make sure I attend – except for holidays or when I'm sick. This hour provides a fixed point in time, a reliable pause, a place to reflect on the ebb and flow of my thoughts and emotions. Some weeks, everything shifts. Other weeks, it feels like a steady rhythm.

March 13th, 2024, feels just like any other Wednesday. I refrain from looking at my notebook – where I usually jot down things I want to discuss – until the end of the session. David immediately notices my pale complexion as I enter, which leads to a conversation about my sleep deprivation, shortness of breath, rapid heartbeat, and the many sources of stress weighing on me. I speak about my past fertility journey and how it still impacts me, and I mention I have a gynaecologist appointment later that afternoon to explore if I have a medical condition. We discuss the heavy stress I am under – from work, family obligations, and the whirlwind of my recent autism diagnosis. David, who typically refrains from giving direct advice, encourages me to take a break from work. While I agree, I'm not fully convinced that I will.

I drive home in quiet contemplation, feeling a mix of relief and doubt about the idea of taking a break. That afternoon feels a little off-kilter. My gynaecologist, though friendly and respectful, startled me during the scan when he said he couldn't see my right ovary. He asks if it had been removed. I explained I'd had a cyst removed in 2011, but as far as I knew, the ovary remained. He gently suggested that it may have been entirely or partially removed during surgery. While I'm left feeling unsettled, he reassures me that my left ovary looks healthy. With a slight smile, he jokingly tells me to have fun this weekend, as I am ovulating.

Despite the levity, I felt tension coil in my chest.

Driving home, my thoughts spiral. Was I foolish to hope for another child? Lost in thought, I missed the turn off for my dad's house and have to double back.

When I finally arrive, I sense excitement in the air. My son is enraptured by the fake jellyfish water lamp my dad has brought back from Australia. The house buzzes with warmth. Dad, clearly jet-lagged, glowing with joy to be home.

After a short visit, we leave. Back home, the evening feels comfortably mundane – cooking, dishes, bedtime routines. At 7 p.m., I sit at my laptop to continue researching the implications of a missing ovary, my thoughts still swirling. Meanwhile, Marek is on the phone with his parents. Then, out of nowhere, he tosses a white envelope onto the table.

I wouldn't have noticed it – just another piece of mail – but something about it piques my curiosity. It has no return address. I open it slowly.

When I see it is from the Public Prosecution Service (PPS), everything else falls away.

Chapter 64: Justice Denied by Design

The first line hits me hard:

"The PPS has determined that your case does not meet the evidentiary standards necessary for it to be brought to court."

I freeze. I hand the letter to Marek, my throat tightening. As he reads it, my worst fears begin to take form. The letter didn't just close my case – it misunderstood it entirely. It misinterpreted my trauma responses as inconsistencies, as if they discredited my truth.

The prosecution outlines how the defence might cast doubt – how the gaps in my memory, the delay in reporting, the nuances of my behaviour, could all be used to dismantle my testimony. What they saw as weaknesses were symptoms of trauma. But in a courtroom, the nuance was lost.

I wasn't the perfect victim.

The PPS wasn't saying they believed I was lying. They were saying a jury might.

And that – that – was the final blow.

For some, justice may look different. For me, it was denied. I could not help but question what kind of justice system allows trauma to be misread as untruth?

Chapter 65: The Friend Who Never Showed Up

"Sometimes the people you love the most become strangers, not because you changed, but because they never truly saw you." — Lalah Delia (attributed)

The letter also confirmed something I had long suspected: that someone I once trusted had not shared information that supported my case. I have already sensed a lack of support, but learning of that in the writing or the absence of the text, so stark and final, makes the loss of our connection feel real in a way it hadn't before.

The "friendship" we once shared – full of memories and shared experiences – now feels shattered. The weight of that loss presses on me, and once again, I feel isolated, just as I did after the attack itself. I just didn't expect a friend to step back at such a critical moment. It felt like a betrayal. Perhaps they had their own fears and reasons, but I've never heard them.

I want to curl up, to scream, to break down. But instead, I go through the motions – helping my son get ready for bed, trying to be present, trying to hold it together.

My mind keeps drifting back to the letter: its cold, impersonal tone. What I want in that moment is my own mother – to feel her warmth, her comfort, her support. But she's gone. And I'm the mother now.

Chapter 66: Bedtime in a Broken World

As I tuck my son into bed, I fail miserably at maintaining my calm front. Silent tears roll down my cheeks; my body is present, but my mind is far away. I cannot shake the overwhelming sense of evil in the world – how rapists walk free, while victims are silenced again and again. Just as I was pinned down, a hand covering my mouth.

Now, with my case dismissed, I will never get the chance to make a victim impact statement. My voice will never be heard in court, and I will never publicly say his name. I will never identify him as the man who raped me.

That chance was stolen from me by a system supposedly built to protect.

The criminal justice system, as I see it now, is designed to protect perpetrators. It gives them freedom, anonymity, the chance to re-offend. It is a system that discourages victims from coming forward. A system that emboldens rapists.

If my insides could speak, they would be thrashing with rage. It took me eighteen years to trust the police, to believe the system might work for me. Eighteen years. Years of therapy, of slow, painstaking healing, to even *consider* reporting the crime.

And now, it feels like all that hard work has been undone.

I am back to square one.

The man who raped me is out there, living his life – maybe preparing for the St. Patrick's Day celebrations. I imagine him smiling, carefree. And I sarcastically congratulate our wonderful criminal justice system for "protecting" us.

That night, I check the locks on the front and back doors repeatedly. Eventually, I retire to bed, my mind a storm of thoughts.

I think again about my missing ovary. The letter. The PPS decision. My belief that the connection between the assault and my infertility isn't a coincidence – the cyst, the surgery, the quiet chain reaction inside my body that no one else seems to connect.

And then, the most pressing question of all: Should I attempt to conceive this weekend?

The gynaecologist tells me that tomorrow and this weekend are my best windows. But how can I possibly make that decision now? What reasons do I have to bring another child into this world – a world so plagued by suffering and malevolence?

Then come the darker thoughts. That friend.

I was heartbroken to learn that a person I trusted did not share certain information with the police that I believe would have supported my case. Discovering this felt like a profound loss. I had always assumed this friend would be there for me, so their silence at that crucial moment was shattering – it felt like a betrayal of our friendship. The betrayal I feel cuts deeper than even the violence I endured that night. Because I never expected kindness or honesty from a stranger. But I *did* expect it from a friend.

I think back to how we once said we'd always be there for each other, no matter what. I quietly forgave their earlier absence after the rape. Throughout our relationship, I gave them chances again and again. But this was the moment I needed them the most. And they chose silence.

Why did I fall for the illusion of that friendship?

The rapist was a stranger. I had no expectations of him. But *a friend*? I did. And that's why this hurt, this betrayal, feels deeper.

Eventually, the racing thoughts slow, and the "big black dog" of depression nuzzles up to me. For the first time in weeks, I feel less anxious. But I don't feel better. I feel heavier. Numb. My body feels like an empty vessel. There's no part of me that can welcome a new life right now.

All I want to do is sleep.

It's this numbness – flat and grey – that gets me through the night.

Chapter 67: The Day the Banks Broke

The next morning, it feels as though I've been hit by a bomb. The suspicious device that once lay at the entrance of Brackenhill Park becomes a metaphor now, finally detonated, unleashing a dam of emotion that bursts its banks.

The flood sweeps over me, carrying with it every moment I've ever felt insignificant, invalid, invisible, or misunderstood. The therapy, the hard-won steps forward – all of it washed away. My trust in humanity shatters all over again. Fear, anxiety, isolation, and rage surge through me like a tidal wave. I am drowning.

Every wound reopens:

The mockery over tartan trousers.
Being left out, only half-welcomed by the girl groups, even into adulthood.
The rape.
The bullying.
The retraumatisation from surgery.
The infertility. The mystery of the "missing ovary".
The cancer.
The death of my mother.
The grief.
The late autism diagnosis.
The drug trip.
The loss of a friend's support.
The maze of the criminal justice system.
The childhood trauma – all too dark to even name.
All of it hits at once.

The adrenaline surges like it did when I was a child, running to the Hilly Field to watch British helicopters land. Only this isn't excitement or awe; this is a sick, shaking, trauma-fuelled torrent racing through my veins. All five trauma responses firing off at once.

Am I meant to fight? Flee? Freeze? Flop? Or fawn?

Just as I was violated by a different kind of flood in 2006 – the trauma that changed everything – I now feel consumed by another. It swallows me whole. To me, it feels like the Crown – the authority that governs this part of Ireland – was absent when I needed protection the most. It failed to uphold the very justice it claims to represent.

I will not be protected.

And neither will others. The man who raped me is free to live and work among us.

It feels like the institutions that claimed to protect me turned their backs.

Chapter 68: The Law Doesn't Care

It's clear the law doesn't care. But I do. Because there is right, and there is wrong.

My autistic traits – my unwavering sense of justice, my black-and-white thinking – rise sharply to the surface once more. I am baffled. As a child, I struggled to understand complex systems, like the British presence in Northern Ireland. It defied logic then, and it does now.

Victims are scrutinised, judged for their reactions. Meanwhile, perpetrators utter "not guilty" or offer only a blank "no comment" and walk free.

There are laws. Rules. And those rules were broken. But the system meant to uphold them seems utterly unfit for purpose.

In a jury-based system, justice is filtered through the public's imagination. Victims must conform to a narrow, sanitised image of what a "real" victim looks like in order to be believed. The system only supports those who fit this picture – those who scream, who report immediately, who break visibly.

But trauma isn't like that. And those of us who freeze, who go silent, who carry on – are quietly discarded.

I now understand: I am not the perfect victim. I'm not the type the prosecution believes a jury will accept. I do not fit the figure they need.

And this feeling of not fitting is heartbreakingly familiar.

Once again, I am invisible. Unsafe. Disbelieved. Crushed beneath the weight of institutional failure. I feel sick, nauseated by injustice, gutted by the cold machinery of it all.

I'm supposed to open my laptop and begin my day. But I can't. Work has become increasingly difficult in recent months, our team shrinking, our workloads growing heavier. And now this?

I call my GP. She agrees: I need time. She signs me off.

In the silence that follows, I'm left facing all that's unresolved. The overwhelm is paralysing. I don't know where to begin. But I do know I need space.

I close my laptop.

I get in the car.

And I drive to my dad's.

Chapter 69: Guilty for Being Me

Reading the details in that letter – the proposed arguments of the defence – I felt cast as the guilty party. As though I had fabricated it all.

There is something deeply perverse in these arguments. Stripped of context and flattened into courtroom palatability, it leaves me suspended in disbelief. How can this be allowed?

I find myself shrinking under the weight of their version of me. A version so unfamiliar, so distorted, that I start to feel paranoid. I begin to wonder if there was always a quiet reluctance to take my case forward. Maybe it was never just about evidence. Maybe it was about who I am.

An Irish Catholic woman seeking justice from a British criminal justice system.

A woman, in a world still skewed by gender inequality. An autistic person – misread, misunderstood, misperceived.

A trauma survivor, whose reactions don't fit the mould.

A delayed reporter, years after the crime.

Each factor places me lower and lower. Each one another reason to doubt me.

I start to ask: Am I believable?

And darker still, I wonder, has rape, in practice, been quietly decriminalised in this country?

They tell me my case doesn't meet the evidence threshold. But what about my trauma? My body language? My testimony? My medical records? All of it weighed against one man's denial, likely versed by his solicitor.

I spiral. Every trauma response fires. My body contracts. My mind races. I move between fury and collapse.

Just as my psychoanalytic journey was bringing threads of clarity, the letter arrived – a white envelope, a silent weapon. The final blow.

A reminder that the justice system was not built for people like me. That the pursuit of justice is obstructed at every turn, even by those who could have shared potentially important information but didn't. That silence, whether intentional or not, still echoes. Perhaps they had their own fears or reasons, but I never heard them. The case was closed without giving me the chance to respond to the defence's distortions.

But why should I have to explain myself at all?

Isn't that what forensic psychologists are for – to translate the incomprehensible language of trauma, to interpret the very behaviours that victims often can't explain themselves?

It took me years of therapy just to understand my own story.

I'm still learning.

The only thing I am guilty of is being me.

Chapter 70: My Casual Shoes on Solid Ground

"Still I rise."

— Maya Angelou

As I turn the ignition, the radio blares the song "Runaway Train". I drive out of my housing estate and onto the main road, cranking up the volume, trying to drown out my thoughts. The lyrics hit me – uncannily mirroring exactly how I feel in this moment.

I wonder, *What if I never go back?* The tears stream down my face as I realise the destination of this short car journey. I'm going to my dad's house – a house we always called Mum's. And right now, I really need to see her.

An essential part of my healing journey was stolen the day she was diagnosed with pancreatic cancer.

The music blares: *"So tired that I could not even sleep, So many secrets I could not keep, I promised myself I wouldn't weep, One more promise I could not keep…"*

As my heart heaves, my gut says something different: all the hard work I've done in therapy *hasn't* been undone. I'm on dry land now. I can breathe through this.

If therapy has taught me anything, it's that I no longer need to run. No more hooks in the ceiling. No more amber bottles full of pills. No more drowning in alcohol. I have David. I have Marek. I have Niamh. I have everything Fiona taught me, each lesson helping me navigate the opposing currents.

Therapy has also taught me to accept the moment for what it is, to allow whatever I feel to exist. My emotions are valid, real, and need to be felt.

So, I let them flow. Just like my tears, they won't last. Tomorrow is a new day.

The following week, I drive myself to the clinic. I park and step out of the car. My casual shoes hit the ground as I walk into the clinic, my body no longer underweight. There is no need for a mask. Not the Covid one. Not the metaphorical one.

I wait for David in the reception area. As always, he greets me with a smile, extending his arm towards the stairs, inviting me to go ahead.

Inside the consultation room, he sits silently, holding the space. I meet his gaze – no eyeliner, no hiding.

I want to tell him about the letter, so I begin the session in so many words:

"David, I'm not the perfect victim."

The analysis, the healing, continues.

Beyond the Story

Closing Words

I have lived as a girl, a woman, an autistic person. I've been a friend, student, mother, daughter, sister, wife, healthcare professional, and patient. I've seen life through the eyes of a victim. I endured trauma and made the agonising decision to report the rape. I fulfilled my duty as a witness, but justice failed me. And in doing so, it failed society.

The man who raped me remains free, his life unimpeded, while I carry the weight of trauma. That alone reveals the system's failure. Rape should never be decriminalised, yet that's what it feels like when survivors are dismissed, and perpetrators walk free.

The intensity of my reactions to the rapist in the years that followed wasn't because I knew him – it was because of what he'd done. Post-assault exposure to the rapist was situational, not relational and yet the proposed argument that the defence may have used was that we were in a relationship.

The system allowed my credibility to be questioned. My trauma was minimised – not just by the man who harmed me, but by others, including the "friend" who could have spoken the full truth and chose silence on what needed to be said. That failure is not mine alone. It affects us all.

Meanwhile, many remain distracted by trivial conflicts – green versus orange, us versus them – while real criminals walk free. It's time to focus on urgent, systemic issues, particularly the silent pandemic of sexualised violence. We need to break the silence and create a society where victims can speak without shame or fear.

The current legal system does not adequately address or understand the complexity of trauma. A jury, as a stand-in for society, needs education. Prosecutors must stop choosing cases based on assumptions about whether a jury can understand psychology.

Too many of us do not fit the "perfect victim" mould. We deserve legal support that reflects the nuances of our experience, not luck. Rape is a crime that often occurs in secrecy, behind closed doors. It should not require an overwhelming amount of evidence to be considered credible. It is unacceptable that, in many cases, justice is only possible when overwhelming digital evidence is uncovered, as happened in the Gisèle Pelicot case. Testimony, trauma, medical records – they *are* evidence. The he-said/she-said model cannot default to his truth. And yet it too often does.

The systemic bias against rape victims needs urgent attention. Fear of wrongful imprisonment should not overshadow the need for justice, and victims should not be judged for speaking out. These issues demand societal and judicial reform.

It is evident, given the statistics, that the attainability of justice for rape victims is obtained through a lottery, but justice should not depend on luck. It should be a right.

If my story resonates, I urge you to support change. Raise awareness. Support organisations like **Advocacy VSV** or **Nexus**. Lobby for change.

This isn't just a women's issue. It's a human one.

Epilogue: A Letter to My Younger Self.

Dear Younger Me,

There are burdens I wish you never had to carry – the ache of being seen but not heard, the weight of shrinking yourself to make others comfortable. The years spent blaming yourself, trying to become the version others expected. The longing to go back in time and talk to the safe people you couldn't recognise then.

You were a soldier without armour, but with extraordinary endurance. I remember how you masked fear with a smile. I see you now beneath that mask. You weren't broken. You were surviving.

Every time you people-pleased, every time you whispered "I'm fine" when you were anything but – that wasn't weakness. It was quiet courage.

If I could sit beside you now, I wouldn't ask you to be okay. I wouldn't rush your healing or hush your grief. I'd simply hold space for you – to rest, to cry without shame, to ask for help without guilt.

I'd tell you that one day, you'll find your voice. You won't have to apologise for who you are. And when you speak, you *will* be heard. Not because you shout, but because you matter.

You will come to know yourself in ways that you never imagined. And when you do, the loneliness you carried will become the very thread that connects you to others.

What once silenced you will become the ink of your story. And the pain you couldn't name – you *will* name it.

You made it. And I am so proud of you.

With all the love I now know how to give,

— *Anna.*

Author's Note

The book you have just read is my Impact Statement – but it is not the whole story. Much of the impact remains known only to me, my therapist, and my husband. From reading this book, you will have seen how, time and again, vulnerability has been exploited. Writing this required balancing the deep reasons for sharing with the need to protect myself. Striking that balance has not been easy.

But there is strength in vulnerability. Strength in choosing to unmask and give voice to what was once silenced. The difference now is that I see vulnerabilities for what they are. I've grown. I'm no longer unaware.

And in that awareness, there is power.

> "I am not what happened to me, I am what I choose to become."
>
> — Carl Jung

Thank you for reading my story.

Acknowledgements

I offer my deepest gratitude to my husband, my son, my family, my therapist and my Godmother, Oonagh. Your love, patience, prayers, and unwavering support have carried me through the darkest chapters of my life.

To the true friends of my past and present– those who remained beside me despite the weight of time and distance, especially Alix, Aileen, Patrice and Colette, thank you for your loyalty and compassion. I hold your kindness close.

Thank you to the McEvoys, it is the smallest gestures and messages of support that sometimes go a very long way. To those who made lasting positive impressions such as some of my school teachers, too many to name, but a special mention to those I've reconnected with in recent times, Oonagh, Briege and John.

To all the professionals who have supported my healing journey, from those at the clinic I attended, the dedicated team at Nexus and Niamh Quinn of Advocacy VSV – thank you for walking beside me.

To my current GPs and medical professionals involved in my care, thank you. I want to acknowledge the care and support many of you have offered me in the most recent years. While parts of this story recounts painful and often invalidating experiences within the medical system, I hope you know that these reflections do not reflect on you personally. Most of the more difficult encounters belong to an earlier chapter of my life. Since embarking on this healing journey, I've felt seen and supported more often than not, including the recent referral to a gastroenterologist, which helped rule out physical causes for what were ultimately trauma-driven panic episodes. That gesture, among others, reminded me what compassionate, curious medicine can look like. I'm truly grateful.

To the women who helped me reclaim parts of myself – sisters Claire and Orlagh of Elysium Wellness, Shauneen Simpson of Heart To Heart Holistic Health and her sister Sarah McCardle of Sarah's Stepping Stones Holistic Health, and Johanne Callan of Try The Alternative – thank you for your care, presence, and insight. And to Linda Murphy of Newry Mums, thank you for managing my anonymous requests with patience and kindness.

To Tony of Leafy Greens in Warrenpoint, and to Angela Martellacci of Il Forno in Florence. Thank you for the warm chats, the laughter, and the kindness you offered without knowing it. Some days I visited feeling weighed down, but your presence, your banter, your food, your humanity, brought light to moments when I thought I had none left. Your small daily gestures meant more than you could ever have imagined.

A special thank you to Dr Helen Williams of The University of Sunderland – who kindly shared her publication: "Testimonial injustice: exploring 'credibility' as a barrier to justice for people with learning disabilities/autism who report sexual violence."

To my editor, Lynne Walker from Glasgow, Scotland. Thank you for helping shape this book with thoughtfulness and respect. Your editing was never just about words; it was about holding the story with care. You worked with the silences, the spaces, and the weight between the lines — honouring not just what was said, but what was felt. This book is stronger, deeper, and more truthful because of your insight and gentle precision.

To Geraldine Walsh. Thank you for providing such thoughtful professional guidance at the very beginning of this journey. Your feedback on my first messy draft helped me see the shape of the story buried beneath the surface. Your encouragement gave me the confidence to keep going. Those early insights stayed with me throughout the process, and I'm deeply grateful.

To Andrea Purdie. Thank you for bringing both the cover and interior of this book to life with such sensitivity and care. Your design work honoured the story at every step, and your seamless communication and steady guidance made the process feel collaborative, grounded, and respectful. I'm deeply grateful for your professionalism, your intuition, and the quiet strength you brought to shaping this book's visual home.

To my advance readers including friends, strangers, and those in between, thank you for reading these pages before the world could. Your feedback gave me the confidence to press forward with publication. This story would not be out in the world without the time you gave to reading and reviewing.

And most importantly I want to extend my gratitude to all victims and survivors of sexual abuse and rape who have spoken out – who have told their stories and sought justice against impossible odds – thank you. Your courage has given voice to others, including me. I stand with you.

And to those who are still silent, who cannot yet speak – I see you, I hear you, and I stand with you too.

You have all helped make this healing possible. You reminded me that my voice matters –that *her* voice matters.

You helped me remove that hand – the hand that covered my mouth.

Bibliography

American Psychological Association. "Trauma." *APA Dictionary of Psychology.* https://dictionary.apa.org/trauma.

Angelou, Maya. *I Know Why the Caged Bird Sings.* Random House, 2009.

BBC News. "Rape Victims' Voices Not Being Heard, Campaigners Say." *BBC News*, https://www.bbc.co.uk/news/articles/c4n1l3n8zg1o.

BBC News. "Rape Victims' Voices Not Being Heard, Campaigners Say." *BBC News*, https://www.bbc.co.uk/news/articles/cn3n3ddlmkgo.

BBC News. (2023, September 27). Northern Ireland: Pre-charge bail limit extended to 9 months. https://www.bbc.co.uk/news/uk-northern-ireland-66942145

Belfast Telegraph. "'I Am Victorious': Brave Woman Watches Step-Dad Tommy Harris Jailed After 'Vile' Attacks." *Belfast Telegraph*, https://www.belfasttelegraph.co.uk/news/courts/i-am-victorious-brave-woman-watches-step-dad-tommy-harris-jailed-after-vile-depraved-attacks/41022364.html.

Brown, Amanda. *No Peace Until He's Dead.* Merrion Press, 23 February 2024.

Chiba, T., et al. "Current Status of Neurofeedback for Post-Traumatic Stress Disorder: A Systematic Review and the Possibility of Decoded Neurofeedback." *Frontiers in Human Neuroscience*, 17 July 2019, article 233. https://doi.org/10.3389/fnhum.2019.00233.

Cazalis, F., Reyes, E., Leduc, S., and Gourion, D. "Evidence That Nine Autistic Women Out of Ten Have Been Victims of Sexual Violence." *Frontiers in Behavioral Neuroscience*, vol. 16, 26 April 2022, article 852203. https://doi.org/10.3389/fnbeh.2022.852203.

Elva, T. (2023, March 27). Thordis Elva discusses why she waived her right to anonymity as a rape survivor [Video]. YouTube. https://www.youtube.com/watch?v=gyPoqFcvt9w

Fricker, Miranda. "Adopting Fricker's Framework of Testimonial Injustice: The Experiences of Sexual Violence Survivors with Learning Disabilities/Autism." *Disability & Society*, vol. 38, no. 1, 2024, https://www.tandfonline.com/doi/abs/10.1080/096875 99.2024.2323455.

Gillen, Sir John. "Northern Ireland Rape Case Review." *The Guardian*, 20 November 2018, https://www.theguardian.com/uk-news/2018/nov/20/northern-ireland-rape-case-review-sir-john-gillen.

Institute for Global Health and Migration. "Learn." *IGMH*. https://www.ighm.org/learn.html.

Kolaitis, G., and Olff, M. "Psychotraumatology in Greece." *European Journal of Psychotraumatology*, vol. 8, supp. 4, 29 September 2017, article 1351757. https://doi.org/10.1080/200 08198.2017.1351757.

Kirkpatrick, K., et al. "A Review of Stellate Ganglion Block as an Adjunctive Treatment Modality." *Cureus*, vol. 15, no. 2, 19 February 2023, article e35174. https://doi.org/10.7759/cureus.35174.

LDN Research Trust. https://ldnresearchtrust.org/.

Lynch, J.H., et al. "Behavioral Health Clinicians Endorse Stellate Ganglion Block as a Valuable Intervention in the Treatment of Trauma-Related Disorders." *Journal of Investigative*

Medicine, vol. 69, no. 5, June 2021, pp. 989–993. https://doi.org/10.1136/jim-2020-001693.

Neria, Yuval. "Functional Neuroimaging in PTSD: From Discovery of Underlying Mechanisms to Addressing Diagnostic Heterogeneity." *American Journal of Psychiatry*, https://doi.org/10.1176/appi.ajp.2020.20121727.

Northern Ireland Executive. *Gillen Review Report: The Law and Procedures in Serious Sexual Offences in Northern Ireland.* 2019, https://www.justice-ni.gov.uk/publications/gillen-review-report-law-and-procedures-serious-sexual-offences-ni.

Petrosino, N.J., et al. "Transcranial Magnetic Stimulation for Post-Traumatic Stress Disorder." *Therapeutic Advances in Psychopharmacology*, 28 October 2021, article 20451253211049921. https://doi.org/10.1177/20451253211049921.

Roberts, A.L., et al. "Women's Posttraumatic Stress Symptoms and Autism Spectrum Disorder in Their Children." *Research in Autism Spectrum Disorders*, vol. 8, no. 6, 1 June 2014, pp. 608–616. https://doi.org/10.1016/j.rasd.2014.02.004.

Saunders Law. "Virtually All Rape Victims Are Denied Justice – Here Is the Roadmap to Failure." *Saunders & Co.*, https://www.saunders.co.uk/news/virtually-all-rape-victims-are-denied-justice-here-is-the-roadmap-to-failure.

Schnittker, Jason. "What Makes Sexual Violence Different? Comparing the Effects of Sexual and Non-Sexual Violence on Psychological Distress." *SSM – Mental Health*, vol. 2, 2022, article 100115. https://doi.org/10.1016/j.ssmh.2022.100115.

The Open University. "False Accusations of Sexual Violence: Research Summary." *Open University Research*, https://research.open.ac.uk/news/false-accusations-sexual-violence.

The UK Trauma Council. "What Is Trauma?" https://uktraumacouncil.org/trauma/trauma?cn-reloaded=1.

Topping, A. (2022, October 5). *Woman sues CPS after rape case dropped when man claimed 'sexsomnia'.* The Guardian. https://www.theguardian.com/society/2022/oct/05/jade-mccrossen-nethercott-sue-cps-rape-case-dropped-sexsomnia

Willsher, Kim. "French Court Acquits Men Accused of Raping Gisèle Pelicot in Landmark Consent Case." *The Guardian*, 23 October 2024, https://www.theguardian.com/world/2024/oct/23/gisele-pelicot-rape-trial-france-court.

Glossary

Term	Definition
Advocacy VSV	A support organisation in Northern Ireland providing advocacy for victims of sexual violence.
Autistic Burnout	A state of exhaustion often experienced by autistic individuals due to masking or navigating neurotypical environments.
PTSD (Post-traumatic stress disorder)	A condition that can develop after experiencing events that are traumatising.
C-PTSD (Complex PTSD)	A condition resulting from prolonged exposure or experience of multiple events that are traumatising.
DSM-5 (*Diagnostic and Statistical Manual of Mental Disorders*, Fifth Edition)	A manual published by the American Psychiatric Association that provides standardised criteria for the diagnosis of mental health conditions.
Masking	The process of hiding one's natural traits to conform to social expectations.
Nexus	An organisation offering support and counselling services for people who have experienced sexual trauma in Northern Ireland.
Neurodivergent	A term used to describe individuals whose brain processes differ from what is considered typical.

PSNI (Police Service of Northern Ireland)	The police force responsible for law enforcement in Northern Ireland.
PPS (Public Prosecution Service)	The legal body responsible for prosecuting criminal cases investigated by the police in Northern Ireland.
Trauma-Informed	An approach that recognises the presence and impact of trauma, aiming to support recovery without retraumatisation.

If You Need Support

If you or someone you know has been affected by the themes in this book, you are not alone. Help is available, and there are people who care and want to support you. You can find support in your local area by searching online. Below are some of key contacts for the UK and Ireland.

Northern Ireland

Advocacy VSV – Newry & Mourne
www.advocacyvsv.com
Phone: 07852 594 677

Inspire Wellbeing – Mental health and addiction support
https://www.inspirewellbeing.org

Lifeline – 24/7 crisis helpline
https://www.lifelinehelpline.info
Call free: 0808 808 8000

Nexus – Sexual trauma counselling
https://nexusni.org
Phone: 02890 326803

The Rowan – Northern Ireland's Sexual Assault Referral Centre
https://therowan.hscni.net

Victim Support NI
https://www.victimsupportni.com
Phone: 02890 243133

Rape Crisis NI
https://rapecrisisni.org.uk/contact
Call free: 0800 0246 991

UK-Wide

Mind – Mental health support and advocacy
https://www.mind.org.uk

Samaritans – 24/7 listening service
https://www.samaritans.org
Call free: 116 123

SurvivorsUK – Support for male survivors of sexual abuse
https://www.survivorsuk.org

NAPAC – National Association for People Abused in Childhood
https://www.napac.org.uk

SHOUT – 24/7 crisis text support
https://giveusashout.org
Text: SHOUT to 85258

Scotland, England & Wales

Rape Crisis Scotland
https://www.rapecrisisscotland.
org.uk
Phone: 08088 01 03 02

Rape Crisis England & Wales
https://www.rapecrisis.org.uk
Phone: 0808 500 2222

Republic of Ireland

Pieta – Support for suicidal distress and self-harm
https://www.pieta.ie
Freephone: 1800 247 247

Samaritans Ireland – 24/7 emotional support
https://www.samaritans.ie
Call free: 116 123

Dublin Rape Crisis Centre
https://www.drcc.ie

Mental Health Ireland
https://www.mentalhealthireland.
ie

Aware – Support for depression and mood disorders
https://www.aware.ie

About the Author

Anna Kahill is a mother and qualified pharmacist. *Not the Perfect Victim* is her debut memoir, born from her experience as a victim of sexualised violence and her journey through a late diagnosis of c-PTSD and autism. After completing the book, she also received diagnoses of ADHD and dyslexia, which continue to shape her understanding of identity and resilience. She has lived in Northern Ireland, Italy, and Switzerland, and now makes her home in Northern Ireland with her husband and son. She finds balance through time with family, being in nature, and exploring special interests such as psychology, music, and creative projects — all of which support her mental health.

Make a Difference

If this book has spoken to you, the most powerful way you can help is by sharing your thoughts. Reviews help other readers discover stories that matter and keep important conversations alive.

Goodreads

https://www.goodreads.com/en/book/show/237535616-not-the-perfect-victim

Amazon

https://www.amazon.co.uk/Not-Perfect-Victim-Surviving-Diagnosis/dp/1068290307

Thank you for taking the time — your voice helps amplify mine.

Printed in Dunstable, United Kingdom

73063730R00131